A Cookbook For Busy Lives:

30 Healthy Gluten Free Recipes

Table of Contents

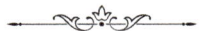

Introduction v

APPETIZERS & SOUPS 1
   Creamy Zucchini Soup 3
   Chicken Tortilla Soup 5
   Chilled Watermelon Soup 7
   Buffalo Chicken Meatballs 9
   Cheese Stuffed Mushrooms 11
   Chicken & Cream Cheese Taquitos 13
   Creamy Coleslaw with Bean Mayonnaise 15

ENTREES 17
   Rice Vegetable & Chicken Salad 19
   Taco Salad 21
   Honey-Broiled Salmon 23
   Roasted Chicken 25
   Rice Noodles with Steak & Vegetables 27
   Rice & Beef Stuffed Peppers 29
   Gluten-Free Carrot Rice 31
   Stir Fry Beef with Orange Marmalade 33
   Salmon Patties 35
   Stewed Tomatoes & Peppers with Chicken 37
   Yummy Polenta Lasagna 39
   Zoodles with Shrimp 41
   Brown Rice Topped with Broccoli & Oven Toasted Walnuts 43
   Mushroom Frittata 45
   Chicken Cacciatore 47
   Vegan Fajitas 49

DESSERTS 51
   Dairy-Free Coconut Ice 53
   Strawberry Frozen Yogurt 55
   Nutty Chocolate Bar 57
   Black Bean Brownie 59
   Apricot and Coconut Balls 61
   Banana Pudding Pops 63
   Gluten-Free Cake 65

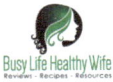

Introduction

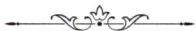

The gluten-free diet is currently a popular diet that can help you in many ways, particularly in reducing weight and the risk of cardiovascular disease. It can also help in increasing your overall energy.

While on a gluten-free diet, you exclude gluten protein completely from your meals which is usually found in grains like barley, wheat, and rye.

This diet is prescribed by doctors and nutritionists to people who have signs and symptoms of celiac disease.

In this book, I have collected 30 easy-to-cook and delicious gluten-free recipes for you. All of these recipes are tried and tested, and I am sure you are going to love them!

Try these dishes and share the love of healthy eating habits with your family.

For additional assistance with transitioning to a gluten free lifestyle, please contact me at glutenfree@busylifehealthywife.com and/or schedule coaching time with me. I have been on the gluten free diet since about 2012.

Happy Cooking!

Monica Anne

©Busy Life Healthy Wife and ©Adventure Reimagined, LLC
All Rights Reserved.

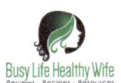

APPETIZERS & SOUPS

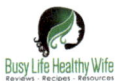

Busy Life Healthy Wife
Reviews · Recipes · Resources

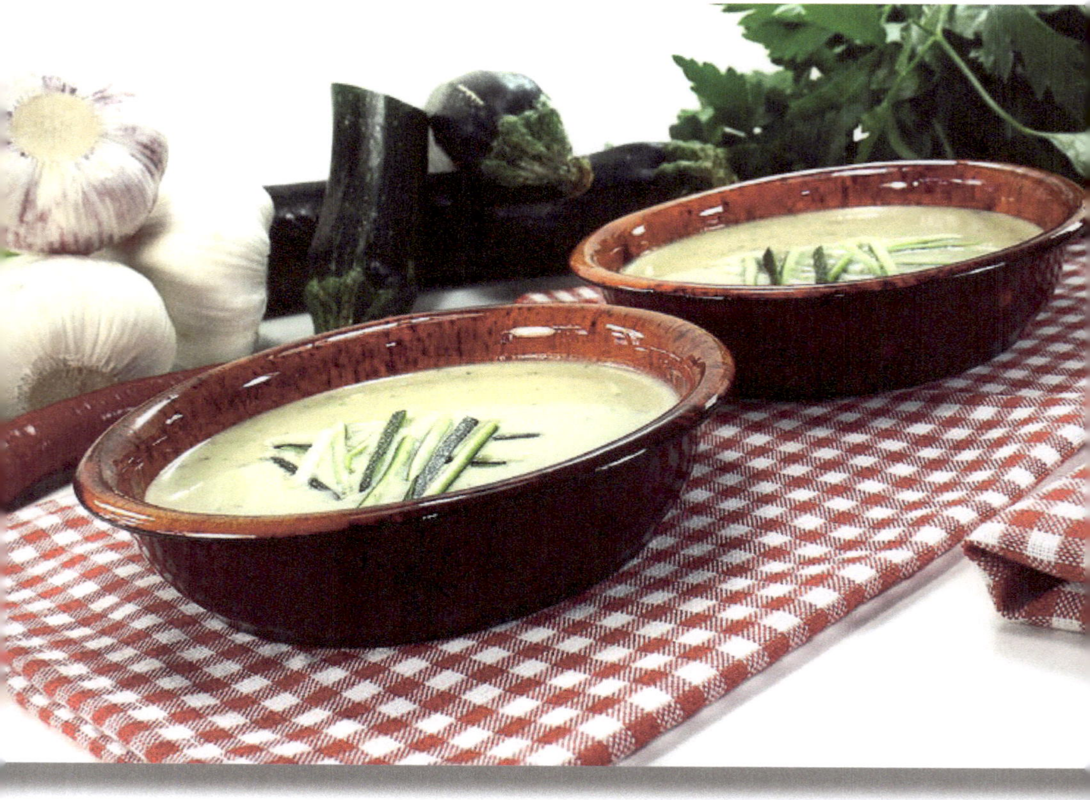

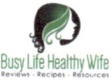

Creamy Zucchini Soup

Serves: 4   Preparation Time: 5 minutes   Cooking Time: 10 minutes

This is a super easy, quick and satisfying gluten-free soup. You can enjoy it hot or chilled, according to your mood and the weather.

Ingredients:

- Zucchini 1 ½ pounds, cut into 1-inch pieces
- Homemade vegetable broth 3 cups
- Fresh dill 1 tablespoon, chopped, or 1 teaspoon dried
- Reduced fat cheddar cheese ¾ cup, shredded
- Freshly ground black pepper ¼ teaspoon
- Salt ¼ teaspoon

Directions:

1. Combine zucchini, broth, and dill in a saucepan and bring it to a boil over medium-high heat.
2. Reduce heat to low and simmer uncovered for 10 minutes or until zucchini is tender.
3. Remove from the heat and puree with an immersion blender until smooth.
4. Return the soup pan to heat over medium-high heat and slowly stir in cheese until it is incorporated.
5. Season with salt and pepper and serve.
6. You can serve it hot or chilled as you like.

Nutritional Facts Per Serving:

- Calories: 105
- Carbohydrates: 9g
- Fats: 4g
- Protein: 9g

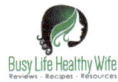

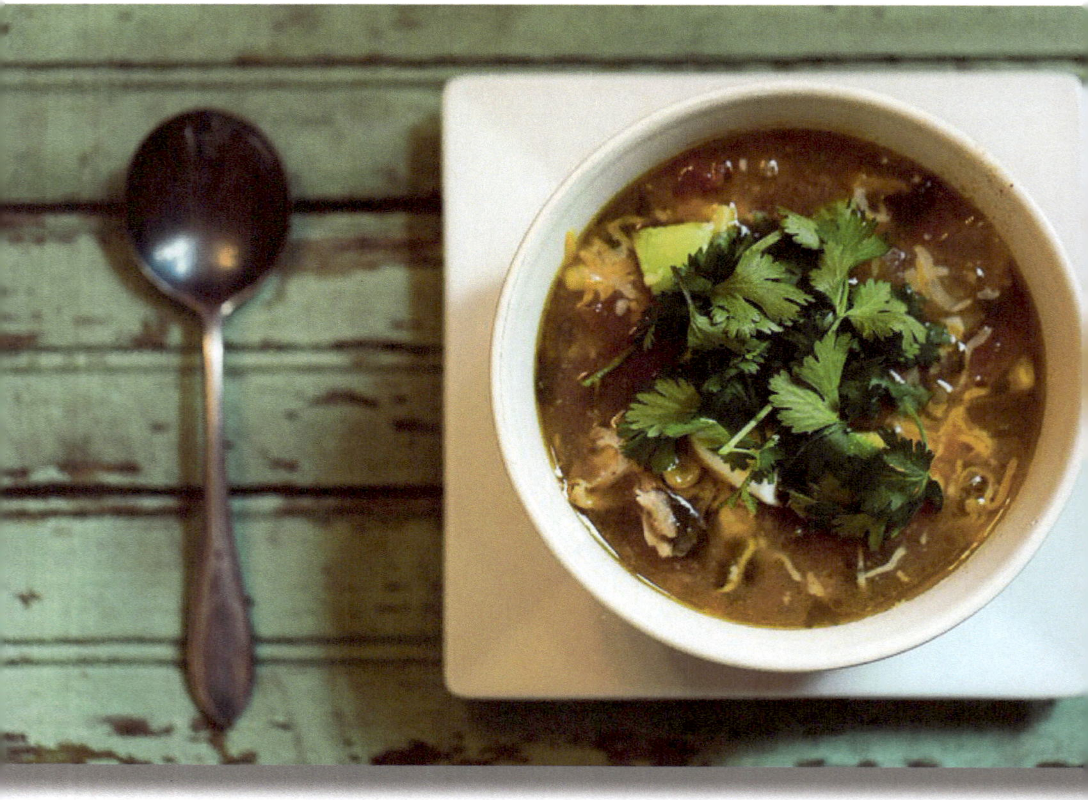

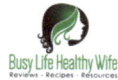

Chicken Tortilla Soup

Serves: 6   Preparation Time: 10 minutes   Cooking Time: 20 minutes

This version of chicken tortilla soup is super easy, healthy, and delicious. You can also use homemade chicken broth.

Ingredients:

- Chicken thighs 1 pound, boneless, skinless, trimmed and cut into 1-inch pieces
- Reduced sodium homemade chicken broth 4 cups
- Corn tortillas 8 halved, and thinly sliced
- Diced tomatoes with green Chiles 1 can (14 ounces)
- Sharp cheddar cheese shredded ½ cup
- Fresh cilantro chopped ¼ cup
- Lime juice 2 tablespoons
- Canola oil 1 tablespoon
- Poblano peppers 3 diced
- Onion 1 medium sized, diced
- Ground cumin 1 teaspoon
- Olive oil cooking spray

Directions:

1. Preheat your oven to 400 degrees F.
2. On a baking sheet, spread tortilla strips in an even layer and coat with cooking spray.
3. Bake for 15 minutes or until browned and crispy.
4. Meanwhile in a large saucepan heat oil over medium heat.
5. Add peppers and onion to hot oil and cook for 5 minutes or until onion is softened.
6. Add cumin and cook for 1 minute, stirring constantly.
7. Add chicken, broth, and tomatoes with their juice and bring it to boil.
8. Reduce heat to low and simmer for 15 minutes or until the chicken is cooked through.
9. Turn off the heat and stir in lime juice. Pour in serving bowls and top each serving bowl with baked tortilla strips, cheddar cheese, and cilantro.

Nutritional Facts Per Serving (1 ½ Cup):

- Calories: 275
- Carbohydrates: 24g
- Fats: 12g
- Protein: 19g

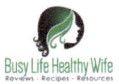

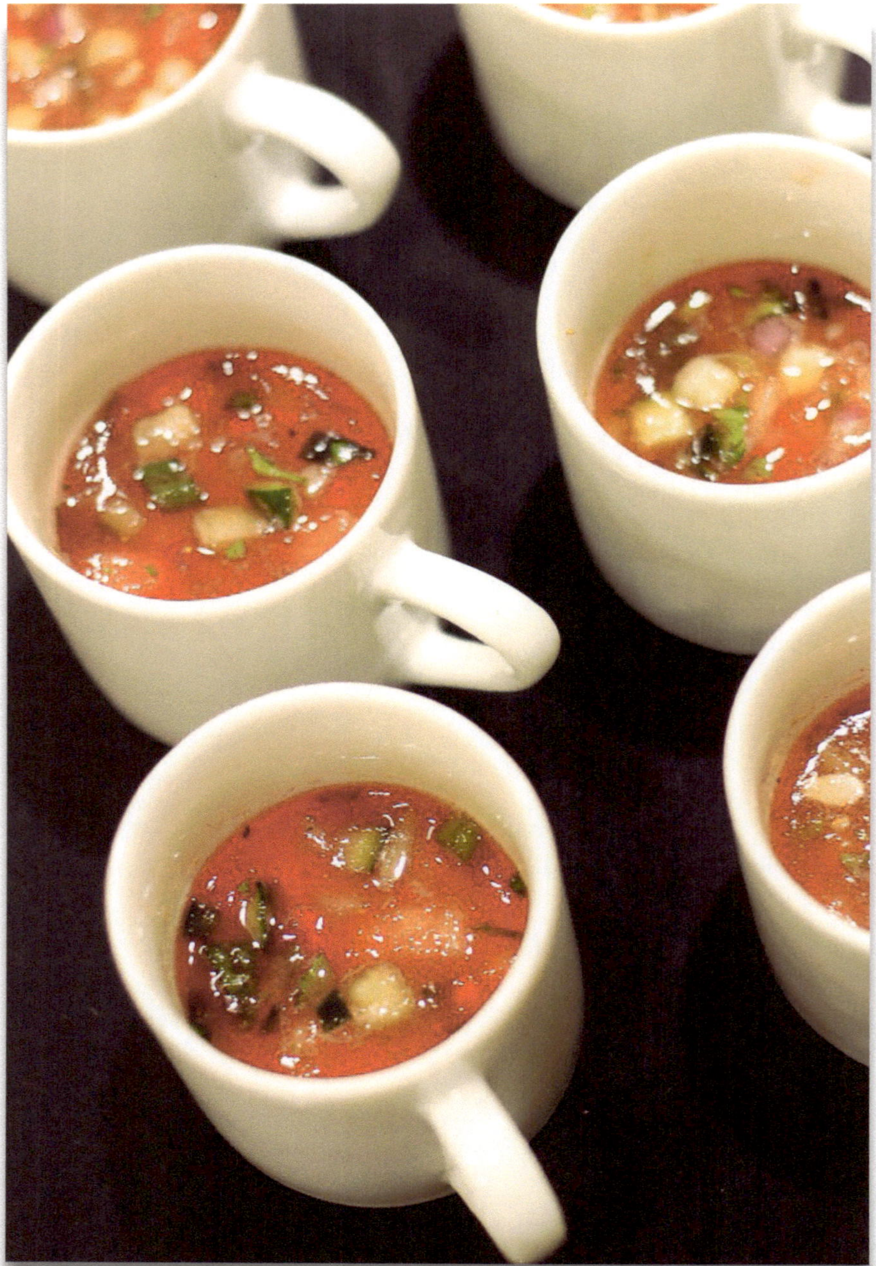

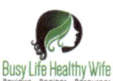

Chilled Watermelon Soup

Serves: 6   Preparation Time: 10 minutes   Cooking Time: 20 minutes

This refreshing soup is gluten free and vegan. It's also a great starter for dinner on a summer evening.

Ingredients:

- Ripe watermelon 6 cups, cubed
- Orange juice ½ cup
- Cucumber ½ cup, seedless, diced
- Lime juice 6 tablespoons, divided
- Cold water 1 cup
- Jalapeno pepper 1 seeded and chopped
- Whole scallion 1 chopped
- Scallion green 1 tablespoon, thinly sliced
- Fresh ginger 1 teaspoon, chopped
- Plain yogurt 6 teaspoons
- Cilantro 2 tablespoons, finely chopped
- Kosher salt ½ teaspoon
- Orange zest of 1 (2 by ½ inch) strip

Directions:

1. Small dice 1 cup watermelon and combine with scallion green, cucumber, and 2 tablespoon lime juice.
2. Cover and refrigerate until ready to serve the soup.
3. Combine the remaining melon, 4 tablespoons lime juice, water, whole scallion, jalapeno, orange juice, orange zest, salt, and ginger in a blender and blend until creamy and smooth.
4. Refrigerate this blended soup for at least 2 hours or until chilled.
5. Then stir in the diced melon and cucumber mixture and divide and pour among 4 serving bowls.
6. Garnish each serving bowl with cilantro and yogurt.

Nutritional Facts Per Serving (3/4 Cup):

- Calories: 62
- Carbohydrates: 16g
- Fats: 0g
- Protein: 1g

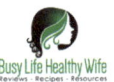

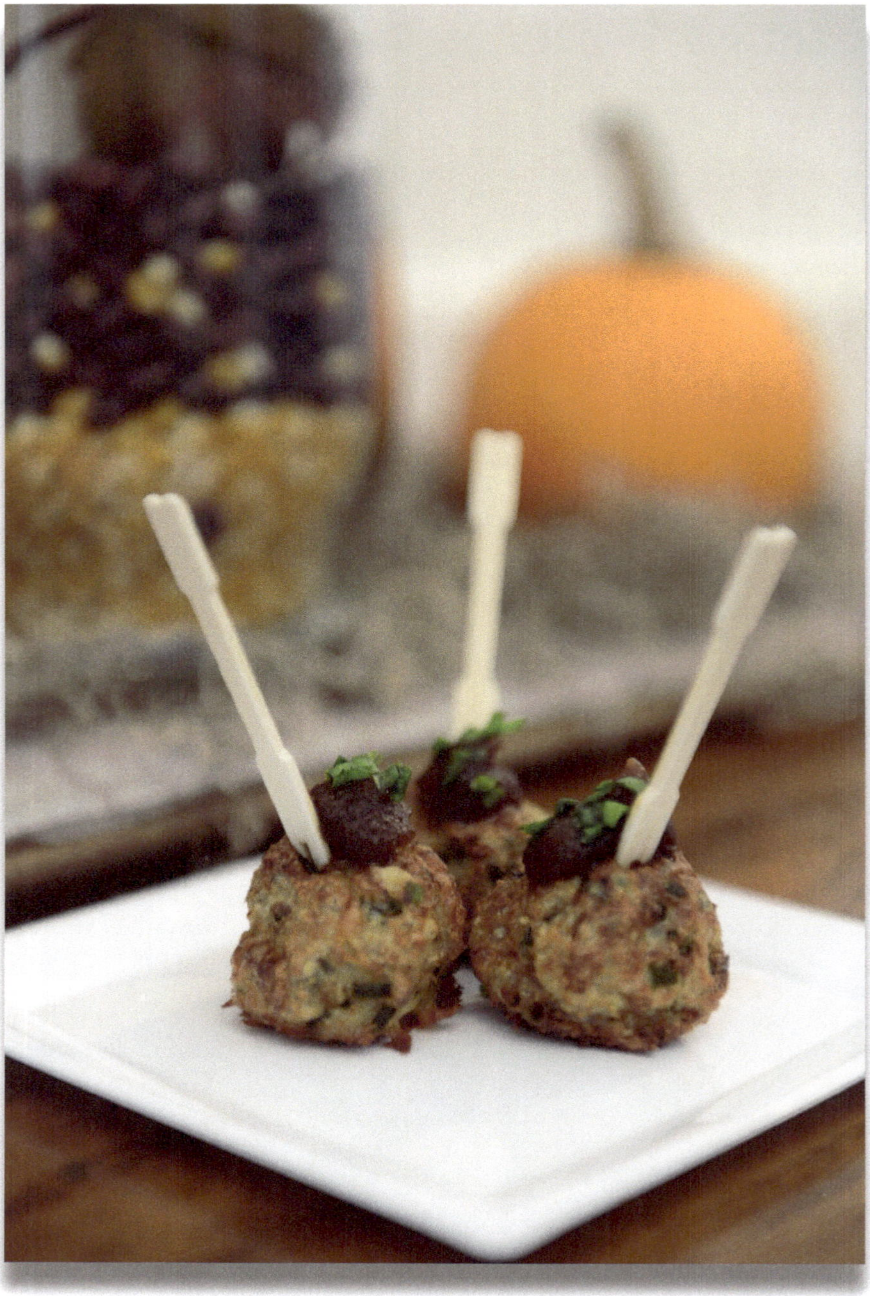

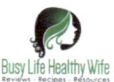

Buffalo Chicken Meatballs

Serves: 14   Preparation Time: 15 minutes   Cooking Time: 45 minutes

These gluten-free buffalo chicken meatballs are a great appetizer and snack. Instead of chicken, you could use turkey, if you prefer.

Ingredients:

- Ground chicken 1 lb
- Oat flour 1 cup
- Zucchini 3 medium shredded
- Egg 1 large
- Buffalo sauce 1/3 cup

Directions:

1. Preheat your oven to 375 degrees F.
2. Line a large baking tray with heavy duty aluminum foil and grease with cooking spray.
3. Shred the zucchini by using the food processor then squeeze excess water with paper towel.
4. Combine all the ingredients along with the zucchini in a large bowl and mix well.
5. Divide into 14 portions and make meatball of each portion with your hands.
6. Place on prepared baking tray and bake for 45 minutes or until they are set.
7. Remove from oven and insert a toothpick in the middle of each meatball and serve hot.

Nutritional Facts Per Serving:

- Calories: 63
- Carbohydrates: 4g
- Fats: 3g
- Protein: 6g

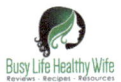

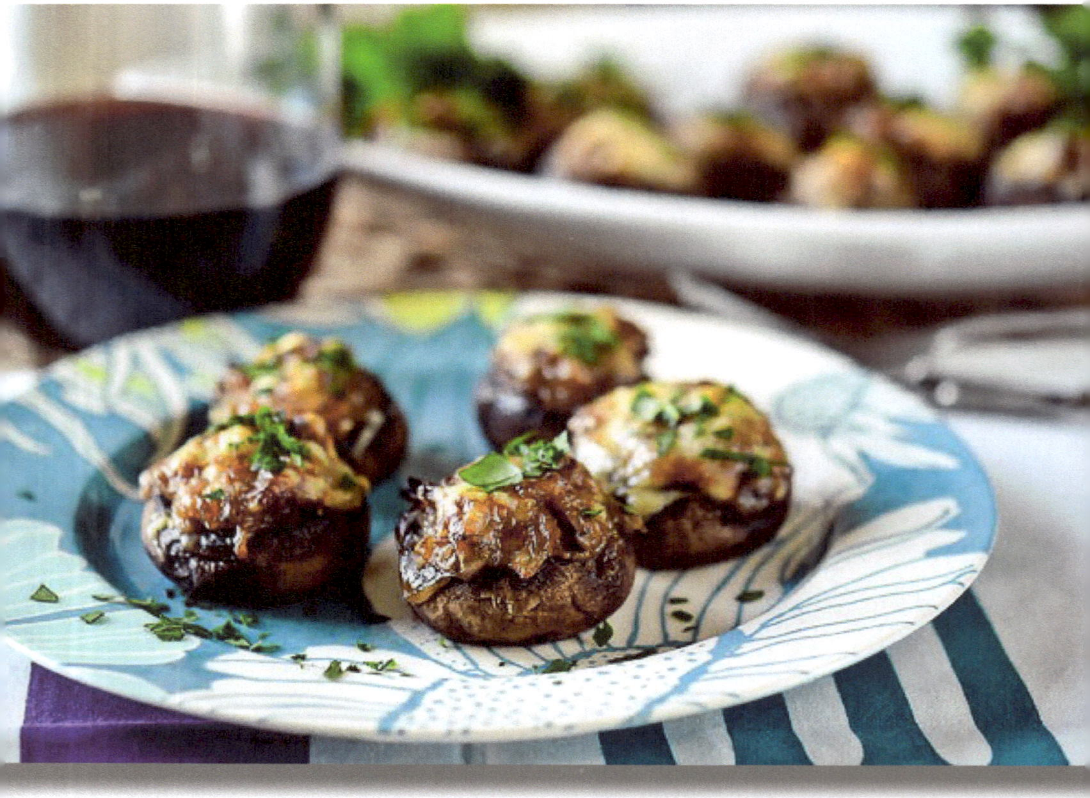

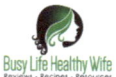

Cheese Stuffed Mushrooms

Serves: 9   Preparation Time: 15 minutes   Cooking Time: 20 minutes

These mushrooms are deliciously stuffed with pepper jack cheese, onion, bell peppers, and olives. (You can always omit the olives.)

Ingredients:

- Whole white mushrooms 36
- Pepper jack cheese grated 8 ounces
- Red bell pepper ½ cup, finely chopped
- Onion ½ cup, finely chopped
- Olives 1 can (4.25oz)
- Double concentrated tomato paste 1 tube (4.4 oz)

Directions:

1. Preheat your oven to 400-degrees F.
2. Clean mushrooms and remove stems.
3. Place the mushrooms in a large baking tray.
4. In a mixing bowl, combine cheese, bell pepper, onion, olives, and tomato paste and mix well.
5. Add a heaping teaspoon of cheese mixture in each mushroom.
6. Bake for 20 minutes or until mushrooms are cooked and cheese is melted and bubbly.
7. Remove from oven let it cool for 5 minutes then transfer to a serving platter and enjoy warm.

Nutritional Facts Per Serving (4 Mushrooms):

- Calories: 38
- Carbohydrates: 1g
- Fats: 2g
- Protein: 2g

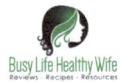

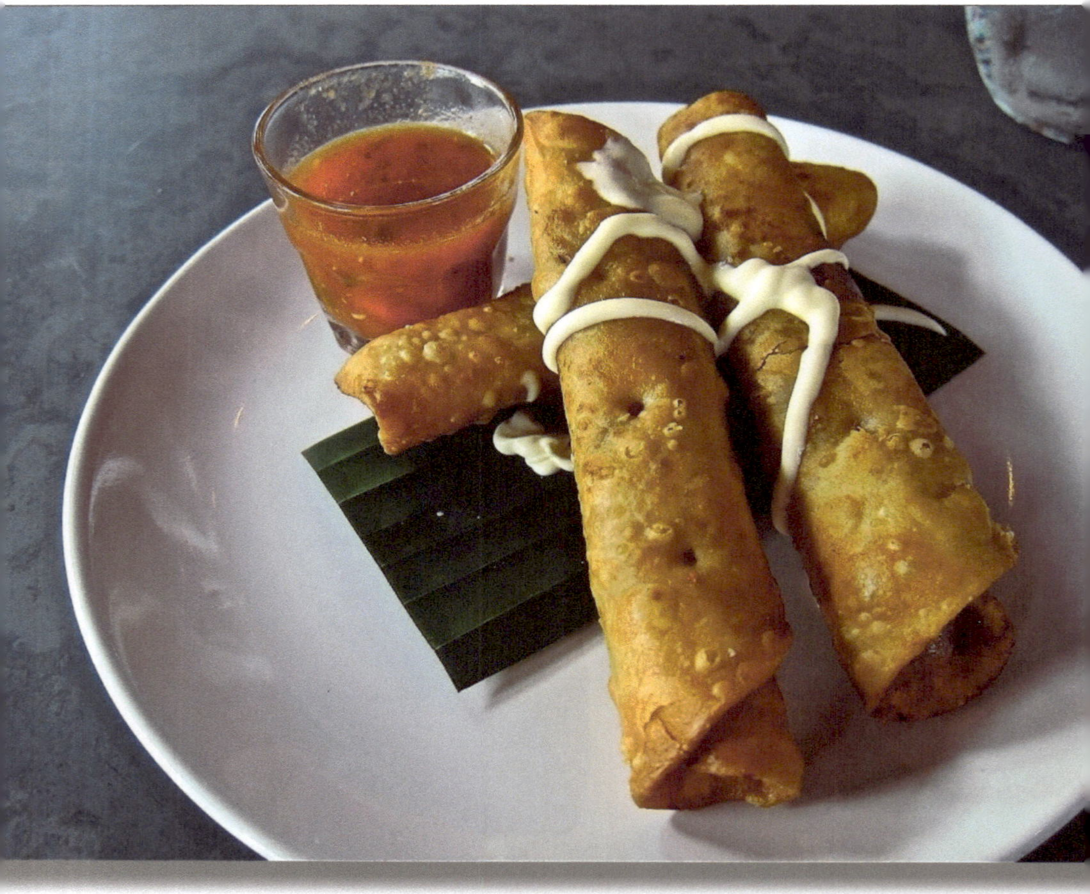

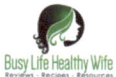

Chicken & Cream Cheese Taquitos

Serves: 12   *Preparation Time: 5 minutes*   *Cooking Time: 10 minutes*

Being gluten free doesn't mean you have to give up Hispanic food. With the Chicken & Cream Cheese Taquitos, corn tortillas are filled with shredded chicken, cream cheese, spinach, and sour cream to make these delicious and gluten-free taquitos.

Ingredients:

- Corn tortilla 12 (6 inches)
- Cooked chicken 3 cups, shredded
- Cream cheese 6 oz, softened
- Colby jack cheese 1 ½ cups
- Baby spinach 1 ½ cups, stems removed and chopped
- Sour cream 1/3 cup
- Salsa ½ cup
- Salt and pepper to taste
- Canola oil for frying

Directions:

1. Fill a skillet ¼ with canola oil and heat over medium heat.
2. Combine the shredded chicken, cream cheese, jack cheese, spinach, sour cream, salsa, salt, and pepper in a large bowl and mix well.
3. Add a few tablespoons of chicken and cheese mixture to the center of a tortilla and spread out.
4. Roll up the tortilla and fry in hot oil until golden brown on both sides.
5. Transfer on a paper towel lined platter to drain excess oil.
6. Repeat the procedure with all the tortillas, fry, and serve warm.

Nutritional Facts Per Serving (1 Taquito):

- Calories: 192
- Carbohydrates: 2g
- Fats: 15g
- Protein: 10g

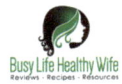

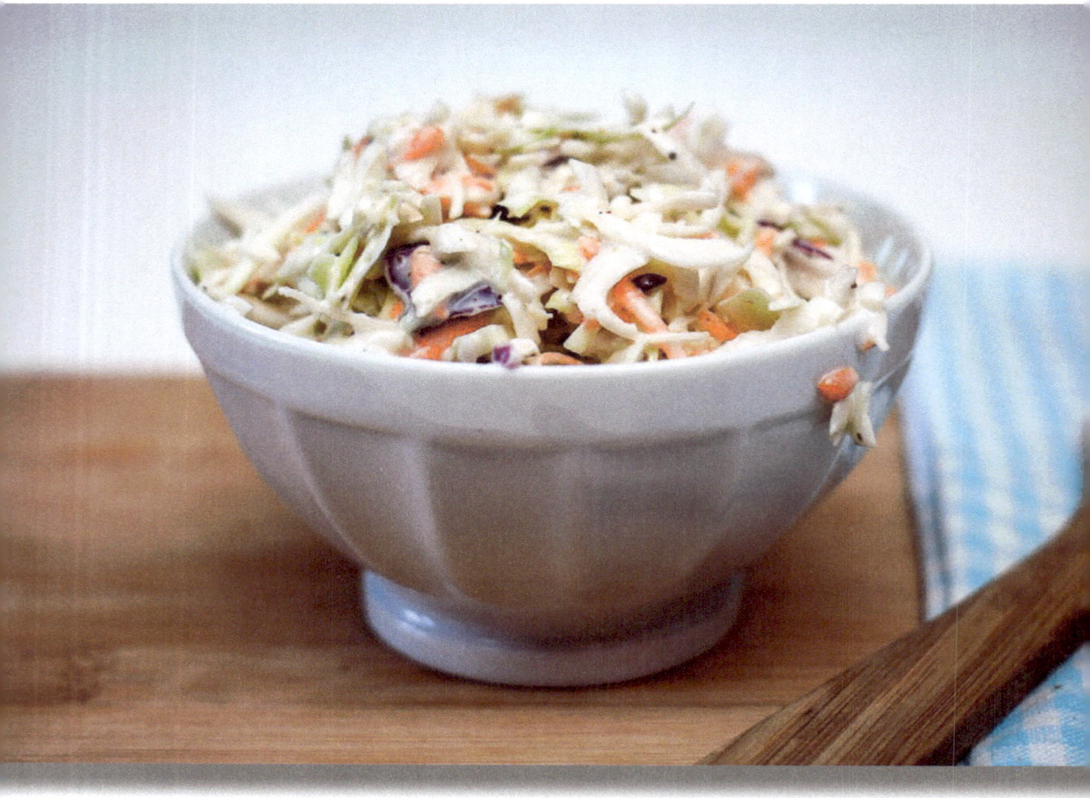

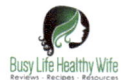

Creamy Coleslaw with Bean Mayonnaise

Serves: 2   Preparation Time: 15 minutes

To make this gluten-free, vegan, and creamy coleslaw, we will be using bean mayonnaise along with fresh vegetables.

Ingredients:

- Bean mayo 1 full batch
- Cabbage green or red 1 head, finely shredded
- Carrots 2 finely shredded
- Red pepper ½ diced
- Yellow onion ¼ cup, finely chopped
- Celery seeds 2 teaspoons
- Gluten-free Dijon mustard 2 tablespoons
- White vinegar 4 tablespoons
- Salt 1 teaspoon
- Freshly ground black pepper to taste

Directions:

1. Pat dry shredded cabbage, carrots, and diced red pepper on a kitchen towel.
2. Place dried vegetables in a large mixing bowl along with finely chopped onion.
3. In another bowl, combine mayo, celery seeds, Dijon mustard, white vinegar, salt, and pepper, mix well until smooth.
4. Pour this mayo mixture in a vegetable bowl and mix well.
5. Taste to check the seasonings add more if desired.
6. Refrigerate it for 2 hours and serve.
7. You can store it in the refrigerator in an airtight jar for 3 to 4 days.

Nutritional Facts Per Serving:

- Calories: 161
- Carbohydrates: 28.6g
- Fats: 1.8g
- Protein: 8.3g

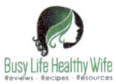

ENTREES

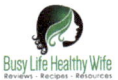

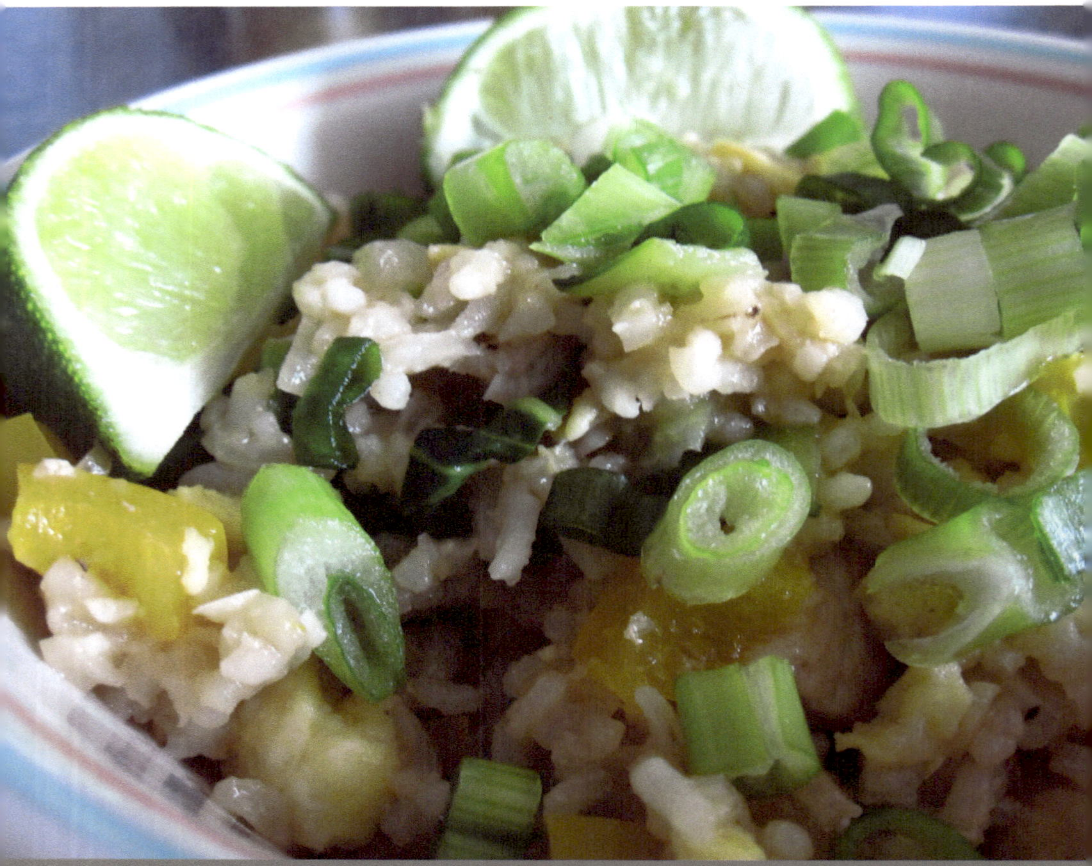

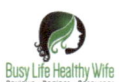

Rice Vegetable & Chicken Salad

Serves: 4   Preparation Time: 10-15 minutes

This is a gluten free and dairy free recipe with a lot of healthy nutrients. Chicken and rice is a household favorite in my home, especially since it's great as left-overs. Note: this recipe is sweet, not savory. Look for savory chicken and rice in my other cook books.

Ingredients:

- Cooked rice 2 cups
- Cooked chicken 2 cups, shredded
- Homemade chicken broth ¼ cup
- Pineapple chunks 1 cup
- Kalamata olives ¼ cup, chopped
- Scallions ¼ cup, chopped
- Orange juice ½ cup
- Lemon juice 2 tablespoons
- Fresh cilantro 2 tablespoons, chopped
- Fresh mint 2 tablespoons, chopped
- Ground cinnamon ½ teaspoon
- Cayenne pepper 1/8 teaspoon
- Salt and freshly ground black pepper to taste
- Extra virgin olive oil 2 teaspoons

Directions:

1. Combine broth, orange juice, lemon juice, cilantro, mint, cinnamon, cayenne pepper, salt, pepper, and oil in a bowl and mix well.
2. In a large bowl, combine rice, chicken, pineapple chunks, olives, and scallions in a large bowl.
3. Add broth mixture in rice and chicken mixture and mix well.
4. Serve immediately.

Nutritional Facts Per Serving (1 ½ Cup):

- Calories: 275
- Carbohydrates: 24g
- Fats: 12g
- Protein: 19g

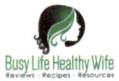

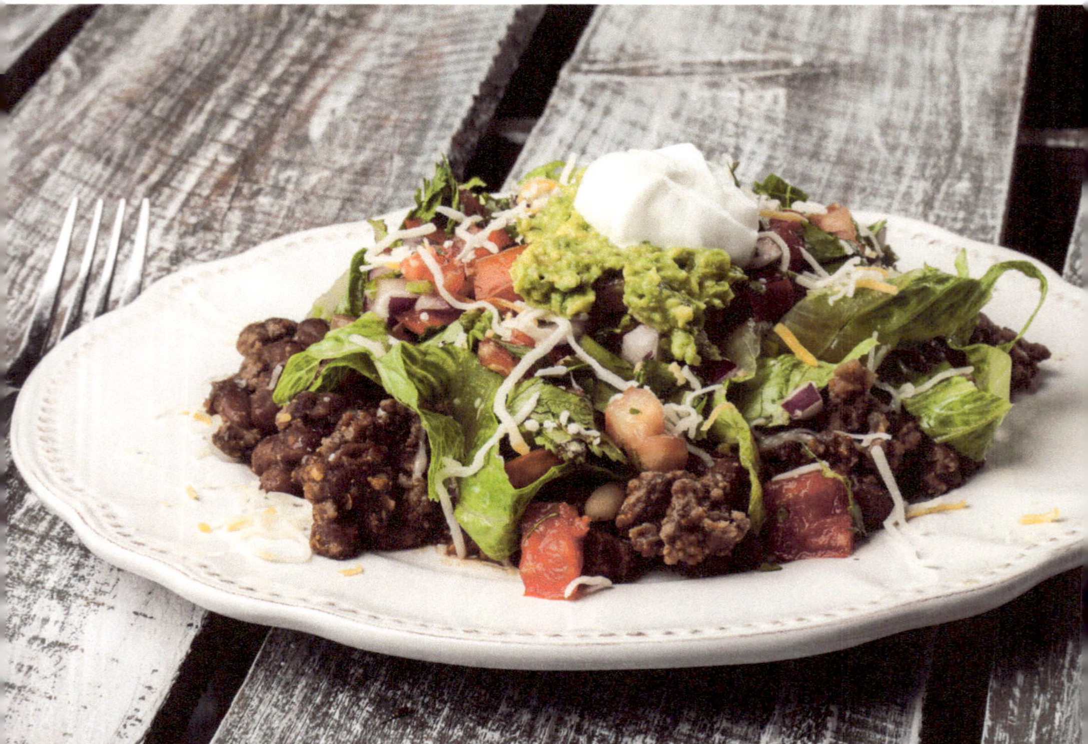

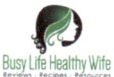

Taco Salad

Serves: 4   Preparation Time: 20 minutes   Cooking Time: 10 minutes

This delicious, gluten-free taco salad is quick and easy to make. You can use lean ground beef or ground turkey.

Ingredients:

- 93% lean ground turkey 1 pound
- Romaine lettuce 8 cups, shredded
- Kidney beans 1 can (14 ounces), rinsed
- Sharp cheddar cheese ½ cup, shredded
- Prepared salsa ½ cup
- Reduced-fat sour cream ¼ cup
- Onion 1 medium, chopped
- Fresh cilantro ¼ cup, chopped
- Garlic 3 cloves, minced
- Plum tomatoes 2 large, diced
- Canola oil 1 teaspoon
- Chili powder 2 teaspoons
- Ground cumin 2 teaspoons

Directions:

1. In a large bowl, combine salsa and sour cream.
2. In a large nonstick skillet, heat oil over medium heat.
3. Add onion and garlic and cook for 2 minutes or until onion is softened, stirring often.
4. Add ground turkey and cook for 5 minutes or until cooked through, stirring often.
5. Add in beans, tomatoes, chili powder, and cumin, cook for 3 minutes or until the tomatoes begin to break down.
6. Remove from heat and stir in ¼ cup of the salsa mixture and cilantro.
7. Add lettuce to the remaining salsa and sour cream mixture; toss to coat.
8. Divide lettuce among 4 plates.
9. Top with the turkey mixture and sprinkle with cheese.

Nutritional Facts Per Serving (1 Plate):

- Calories: 477
- Carbohydrates: 27g
- Fats: 19g
- Protein: 42g

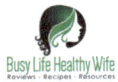

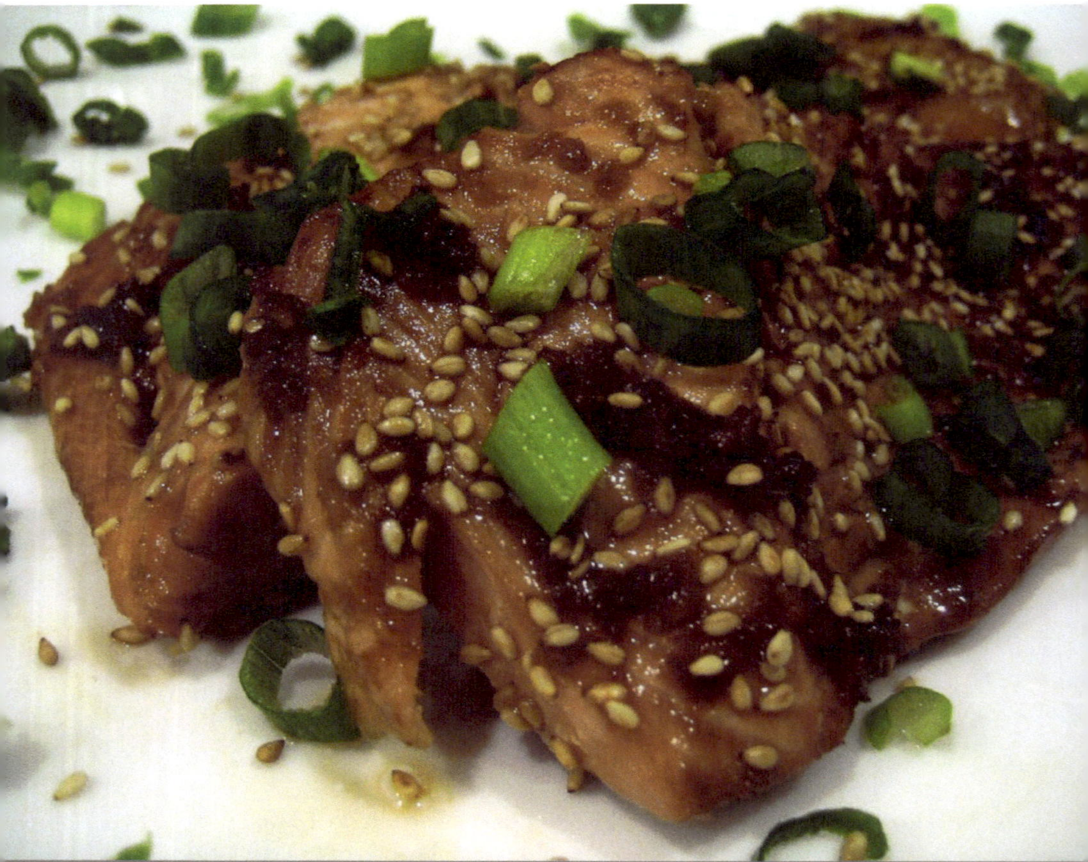

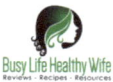

Honey-Broiled Salmon

Serves: 4   Preparation Time: 10 minutes   Cooking Time: 10 minutes

This is a fast and easy way to prepare a classic, delicious, and gluten-free salmon main dish.

Ingredients:

- Center cut salmon fillet 1 pound, skinned and cut into 4 portions
- Gluten-free soy sauce, 2 tablespoons
- Honey, 1 tablespoon
- Rice vinegar, 1 tablespoon
- Scallion, 1 minced
- Fresh ginger, 1 teaspoon, minced
- Toasted sesame seeds, 1 teaspoon

Directions:

1. In a medium bowl, whisk together scallion, honey, soy sauce, vinegar, and ginger until the honey is dissolved.
2. Place salmon in a zip-loc bag, add 3 tablespoons of honey sauce into the bag zip-loc the bag and refrigerate for 15 minutes, reserve the remaining honey sauce.
3. Preheat your oven's broiler.
4. Line a baking pan with aluminum foil and lightly coat with cooking spray.
5. Transfer the salmon to prepared baking pan, skinned side down, discard the marinade.
6. Broil the salmon 6 inches from the heat source for 8 to 10 minutes or until cooked through.
7. Remove from the oven, drizzle with the remaining honey sauce and garnish with the sesame seeds.

Nutritional Facts Per Serving (1 ½ Cup):

- Calories: 160
- Carbohydrates: 6g
- Fats: 5g
- Protein: 23g

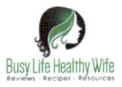

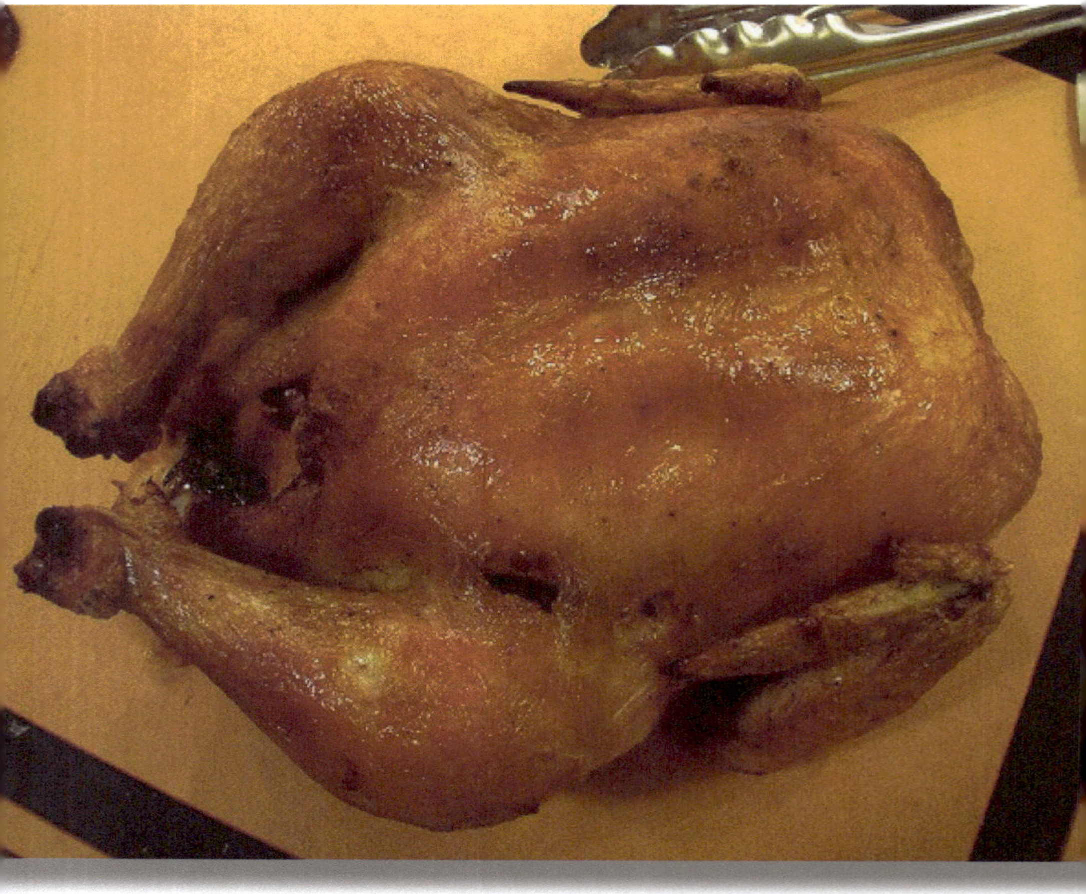

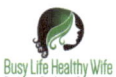

Roasted Chicken

Serves: 6   Preparation Time: 10 minutes   Cooking Time: 1 hour 15 minutes

This delish roasted chicken is so simple, juicy, and made with only five ingredients.

Ingredients:
- Whole chicken 1 (3 pounds), giblets removed
- Margarine ½ cup, divided
- Celery 1 stalk, leaves removed
- Onion powder 1 tablespoon
- Salt and pepper to taste

Directions:
1. Preheat your oven to 350 degrees F.
2. In a roasting pan, place chicken and generously season inside and out with salt and pepper.
3. Sprinkle inside and out with onion powder.
4. Place 3 tablespoon in the chicken cavity.
5. Arrange dollops of the remaining margarine around the chicken's exterior.
6. Cut the celery into 4 pieces and place in the chicken cavity.
7. Bake for 1 hour 15 minutes, uncovered.
8. Remove chicken from oven and baste with melted margarine and drippings, cover the chicken with aluminum foil and allow to rest for 30 minutes before serving.

Nutritional Facts Per Serving:
- Calories: 423
- Carbohydrates: 1.2g
- Fats: 32.1g
- Protein: 30.9g

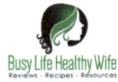

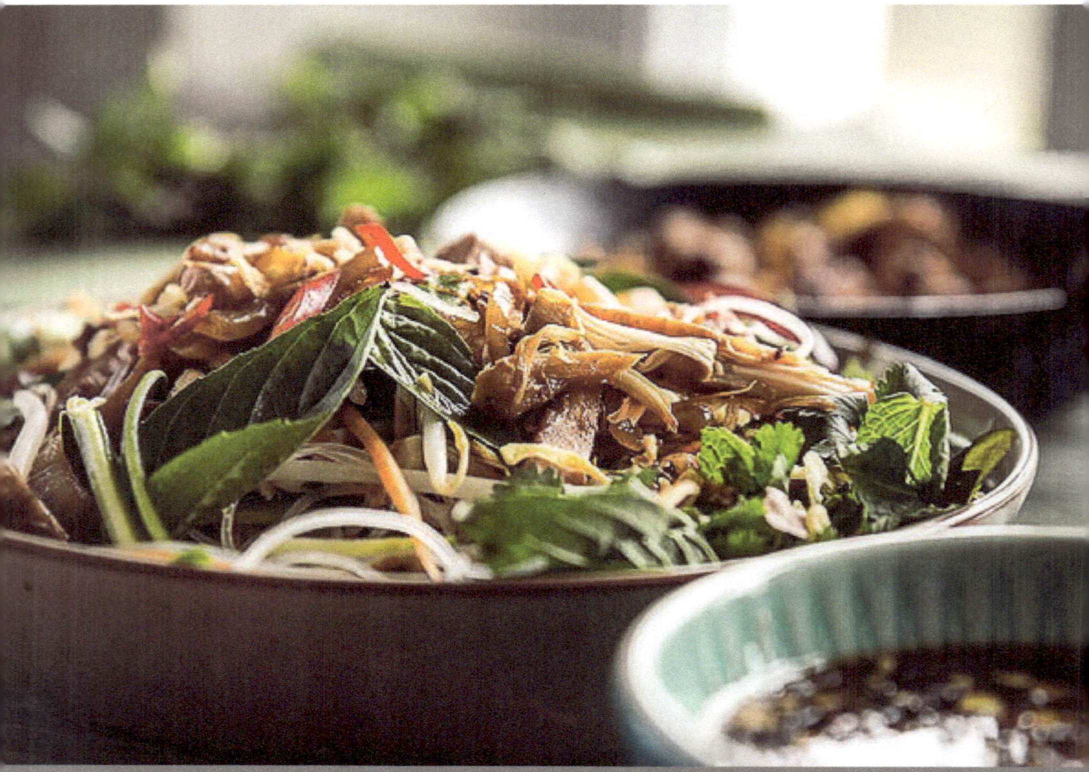

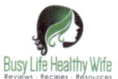

Rice Noodles with Steak & Vegetables

Serves: 6   Preparation Time: 20 minutes   Cooking Time: 10 minutes

In this tempting recipe, rice noodles are tossed with thinly sliced steak, vegetables, and fish sauce.

Ingredients:

- Sirloin steak 1 pound
- Wide rice noodles 6 ounces
- Napa cabbage 4 cups, shredded
- Carrot 1 ½ cups, shredded
- Radishes 1 cup, thinly sliced
- Fresh basil or mint 1 cup, slivered
- Rice vinegar ½ cup
- Sugar 2 tablespoons
- Fish sauce 2 tablespoons
- Canola oil 1 tablespoon
- Unsalted roasted peanuts ½ cup, finely chopped

Directions:

1. In a large cast iron skillet, heat oil over medium-high heat until shimmering.
2. Add steak, reduce heat to medium and cook for 5 minutes per side.
3. Transfer steak onto a clean cutting board and let it rest for 5 minutes.
4. Meanwhile, cook noodles according to package direction, drain, and rinse under cold water.
5. In a large bowl, add fish sauce, vinegar, and sugar and whisk well until sugar is completely dissolved.
6. Slice the steak into thin matchsticks.
7. Add the steak and any accumulated juice to the bowl.
8. Add in noodles, veggies, basil/or mint, and peanuts and toss to combine.
9. Serve immediately.

Nutritional Facts Per Serving (1 ½ Cup):

- Calories: 343
- Carbohydrates: 39g
- Fats: 12g
- Protein: 21g

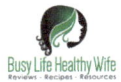

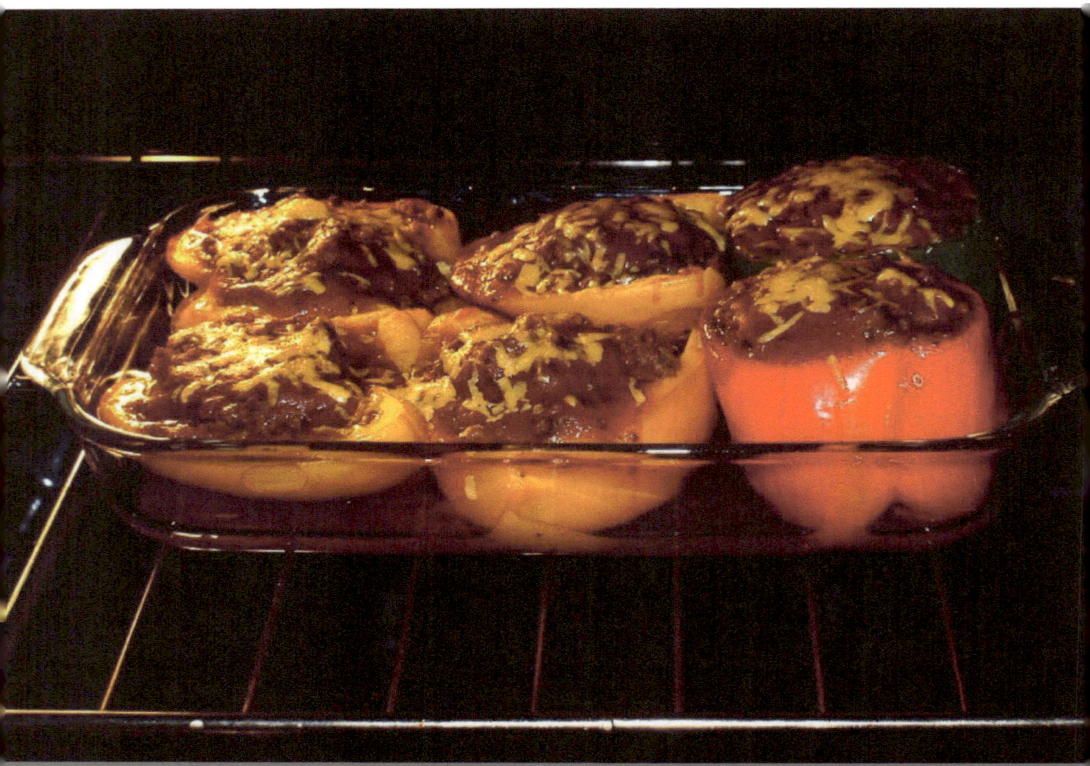

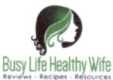

Rice & Beef Stuffed Peppers

Serves: 6   Preparation Time: 20 minutes   Cooking Time: 1 hour

These tempting and delicious bell peppers are stuffed with cooked rice and beef and topped with seasoned tomato sauce.

Ingredients:

- Bell peppers 6 large, tops removed, seeded (you can use any color)
- Uncooked long grain white rice ½ cup
- Ground beef 1 pound
- Water 1 cup
- Tomato sauce 2 (8 ounces) cans
- Homemade Worcestershire sauce 1 tablespoon
- Italian seasoning 1 teaspoon
- Garlic powder ¼ teaspoon
- Onion powder ¼ teaspoon
- Shredded cheddar cheese ¼ cup
- Salt and freshly ground black pepper to taste

Directions:

1. Preheat your oven to 175 degrees C (350 degrees F).
2. Combine rice and water in a pan and bring to a boil over high heat.
3. Reduce heat to medium-low, cover, and cook for 20 minutes or until completely done.
4. Cook beef in a skillet over medium heat until evenly browned.
5. In a baking dish, arrange the peppers with the hollowed side facing upward.
6. Combine cooked rice, beef, 1 can tomato sauce, garlic powder, onion powder, Worcestershire sauce, pepper, and salt in a bowl and mix well.
7. Spoon an equal amount of rice and beef mixture into each pepper.
8. In a bowl, combine remaining tomato sauce and Italian seasoning and mix well. Evenly distribute this tomato sauce mixture over peppers.
9. Top each bell pepper with shredded cheese. Bake 1 hour or until the peppers are tender in the preheated oven, basting with sauce every 15 minutes.

Nutritional Facts Per Serving (1 Pepper):

- Calories: 254
- Carbohydrates: 26.6g
- Fats: 9.6g
- Protein: 18g

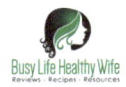

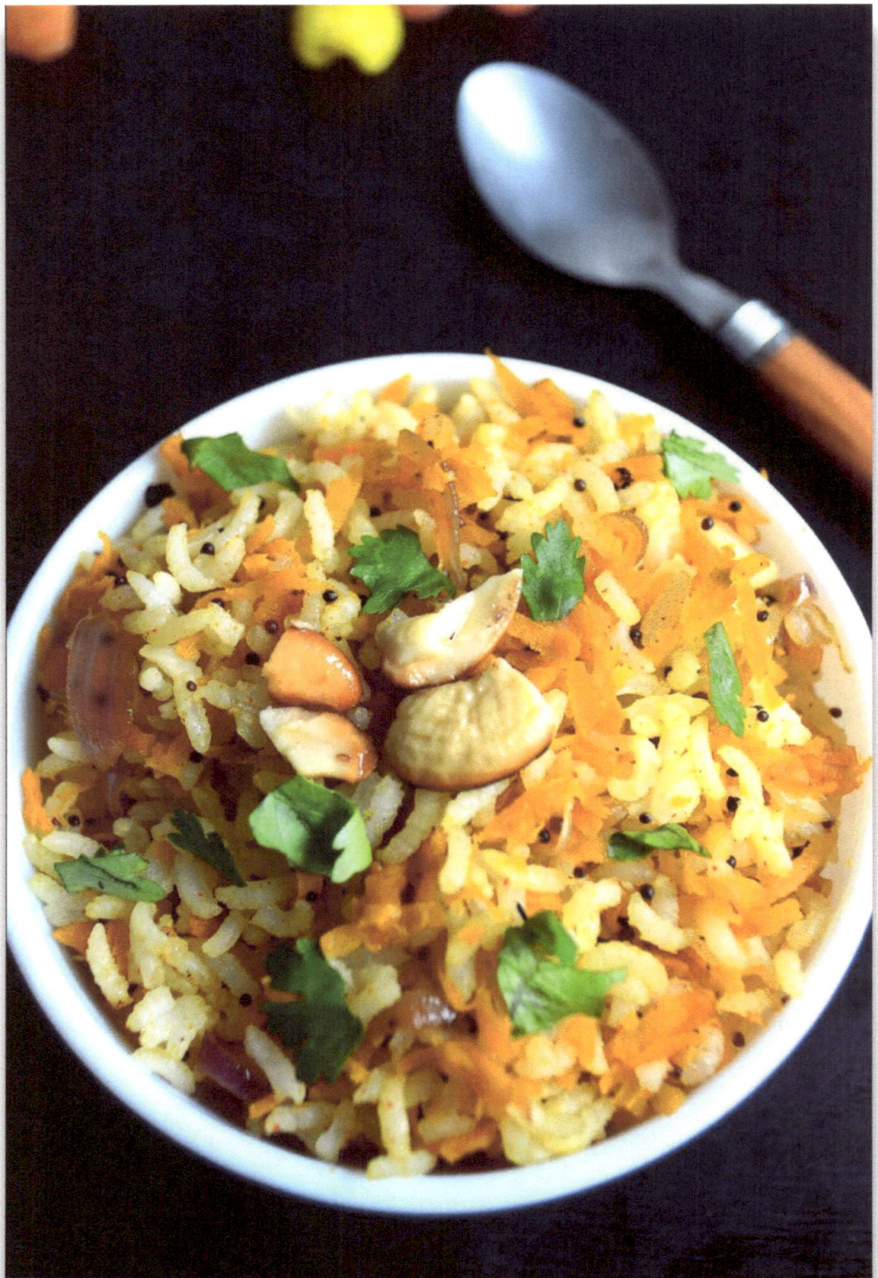

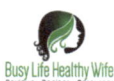

Gluten-Free Carrot Rice

Serves: 6   Preparation Time: 15 minutes   Cooking Time: 20 minutes

Grated carrots are cooked with butter and peanuts, seasoned with cayenne pepper then mixed with white rice.

Ingredients:

- Long grain white rice 1 cup
- Water 2 cups
- Grated carrots ¾ cup
- Onion 1 sliced
- Fresh ginger root 1 teaspoon, minced
- Roasted peanuts ¼ cup
- Margarine 1 tablespoon
- Cayenne pepper to taste
- Salt and pepper to taste
- Fresh cilantro chopped, for garnish

Directions:

1. Bring water and rice to a boil in a medium sauce pan over high heat.
2. Reduce heat to low, cover and cook for 20 minutes or until tender.
3. Meanwhile, grind peanuts in a blender and set aside.
4. In a skillet, melt the margarine over medium heat, add onion and cook for 10 minutes or until it turned lightly golden brown.
5. Stir in ginger, salt, and grated carrots.
6. Reduce heat to low, cover to steam for 5 minutes.
7. Then stir in cayenne pepper and peanuts.
8. Add cooked rice to skillet and stir gently to combine with other ingredients.
9. Garnish with fresh chopped cilantro and serve.

Nutritional Facts Per Serving:

- Calories: 179
- Carbohydrates: 31.8g
- Fats: 4.8g
- Protein: 4g

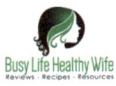

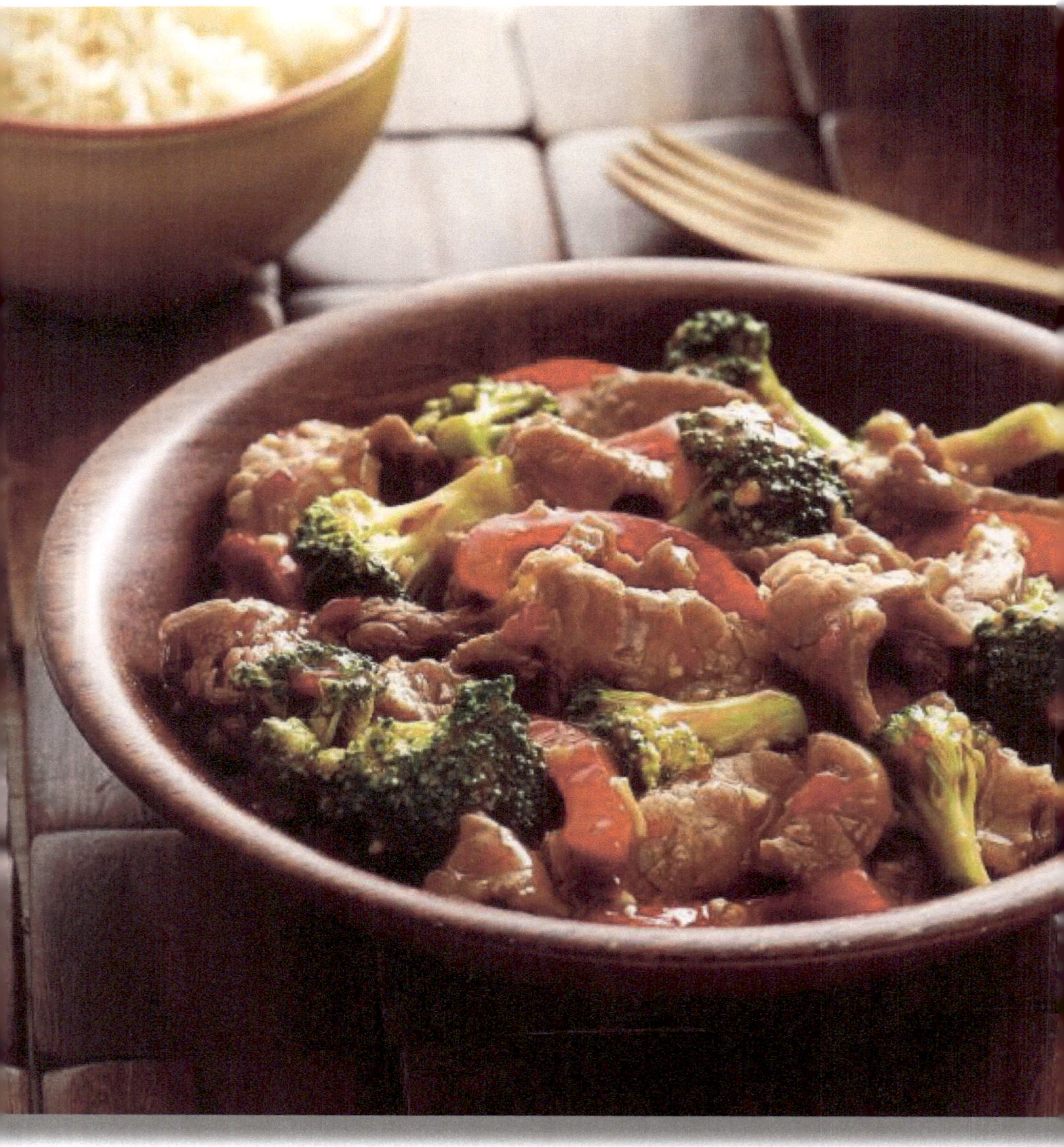

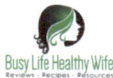

Stir Fry Beef with Orange Marmalade

Serves: 4   Preparation Time: 10 minutes   Cooking Time: 10 minutes

This stir fry beef is easy to make. Orange marmalade is the secret ingredient in this quick recipe.

Ingredients:

- Beef top sirloin 12 ounces, trimmed of fat and cut into ¼ inch strips
- Homemade chicken broth ½ cup, divided
- Broccoli florets 1 pound (4 cups)
- Onion 1 large slivered
- Red bell pepper 1 small, diced
- Fresh ginger 1 tablespoon, minced
- Orange marmalade 2 tablespoons
- Gluten-free soy sauce 2 tablespoons
- Rice vinegar 1 tablespoon
- Oyster flavored sauce 1 tablespoon
- Corn starch 1 tablespoon
- Chili-garlic sauce 2 teaspoons
- Canola oil 4 teaspoons

Directions:

1. In a bowl, mix together ¼ cup broth, marmalade, soy sauce, vinegar, oyster sauce, chili garlic sauce, and cornstarch.
2. In a large nonstick wok or skillet, heat 2 teaspoons of oil over high heat.
3. Add the beef and stir fry for 4 minutes or until browned, transfer to a plate.
4. Add the remaining 2 teaspoons of oil to the wok and add ginger, stir fry for 30 seconds or until fragrant.
5. Add onion and stir fry for 30 seconds.
6. Then add broccoli florets and stir fry for 30 more seconds.
7. Pour in the remaining ¼ cup broth, cover and cook for 3 to 4 minutes or until the vegetables are crisp-tender.
8. Push the vegetables to the side of the wok and add in the corn starch mixture, stir continuously until sauce becomes translucent and thick.
9. Stir the vegetables into the sauce and return the beef to the wok.
10. Toss to coat and serve immediately.

Nutritional Facts Per Serving (1 ¼ Cup):

- Calories: 265
- Carbohydrates: 23g
- Fats: 11g
- Protein: 20g

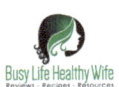

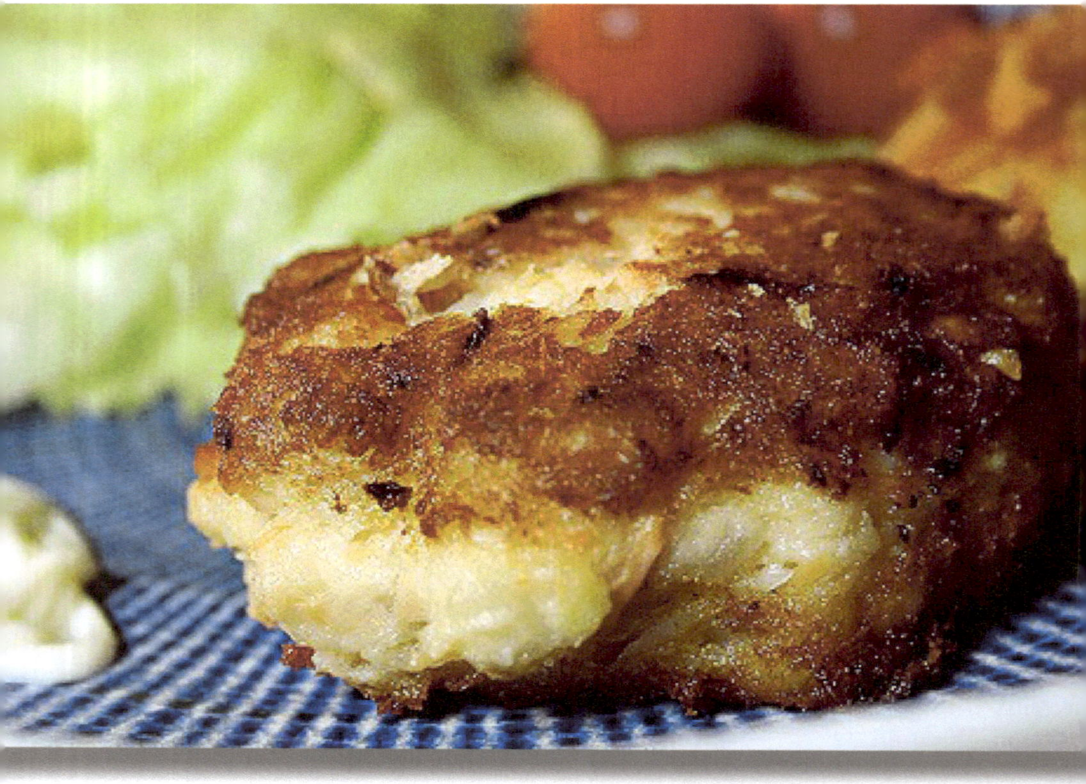

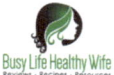

Salmon Patties

Serves: 4   Preparation Time: 10 minutes   Cooking Time: 20 minutes

Salmon patties are not only delicious but also easy to make. You can serve it with salad, sautéed vegetables, or gluten free macaroni and cheese.

Ingredients:

- Salmon 1 can (14.75 ounces), drained, bones removed and flaked
- Onion 1 small diced
- Eggs 2 beaten
- Vegetable oil 3 tablespoons
- Ground black pepper 1 teaspoon

Directions:

1. Combine salmon, onion, eggs, and pepper in a bowl and mix well.
2. Shape into 2-ounce patties; it will make about 8 patties.
3. Heat the oil in a large skillet over medium heat.
4. Fry each patty about 5 minutes per side or until golden and crispy.

Nutritional Facts Per Serving (2 Patties):

- Calories: 307
- Carbohydrates: 2.3g
- Fats: 20.3g
- Protein: 27.5g

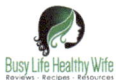

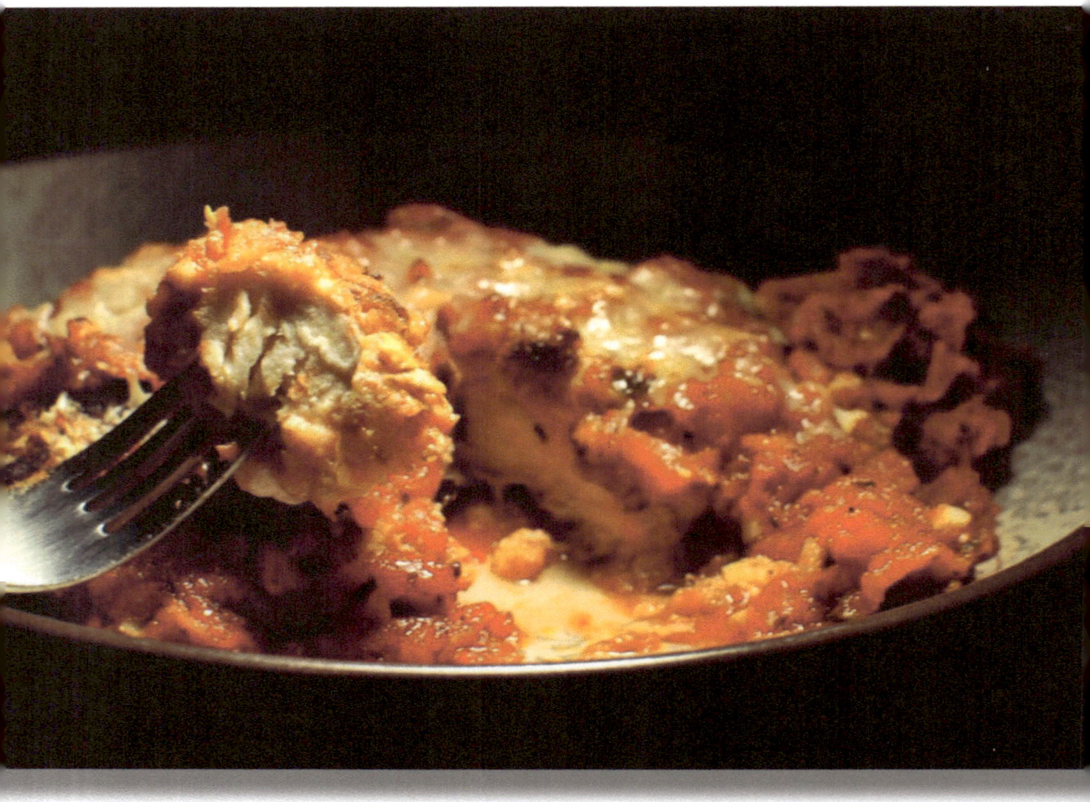

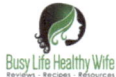

Stewed Tomatoes & Peppers with Chicken

Serves: 4   Preparation Time: 5 minutes   Cooking Time: 20 minutes

Tomatoes, peppers, and onion are first stewed with chicken on the stove then roasted in the oven. It gives the chicken a unique flavor that your family will love.

Ingredients:

- Large cherry tomatoes ½ lbs, halved
- Red bell pepper 2 quartered and sliced crosswise ½ inch thick
- Red onion 2 small, cut into ½ inch thick wedges
- Garlic 2 cloves, thinly sliced
- Chicken breasts 4 (6 oz each), boneless, skinless
- Olive oil 1 tablespoon
- Smoked paprika 1 tablespoon
- Kosher salt and pepper to taste
- Parsley and sliced almonds, for serving

Directions:

1. Heat your oven to 450 degrees F.
2. With a paper towel pat dry chicken.
3. Rub chicken with paprika, salt, and pepper.
4. In a large skillet, heat oil over medium heat and cook chicken for 5 minutes on one side or until browned.
5. Turn chicken over and add garlic, bell pepper, onion, and tomato to the skillet.
6. Season with salt and pepper.
7. Transfer skillet to preheated oven and roast for 14 minutes or until chicken and vegetables are tender.
8. Remove from oven sprinkle parsley and sliced almonds and serve.

Nutritional Facts Per Serving:

- Calories: 285
- Carbohydrates: 11g
- Fats: 8.5g
- Protein: 40g

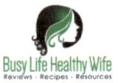

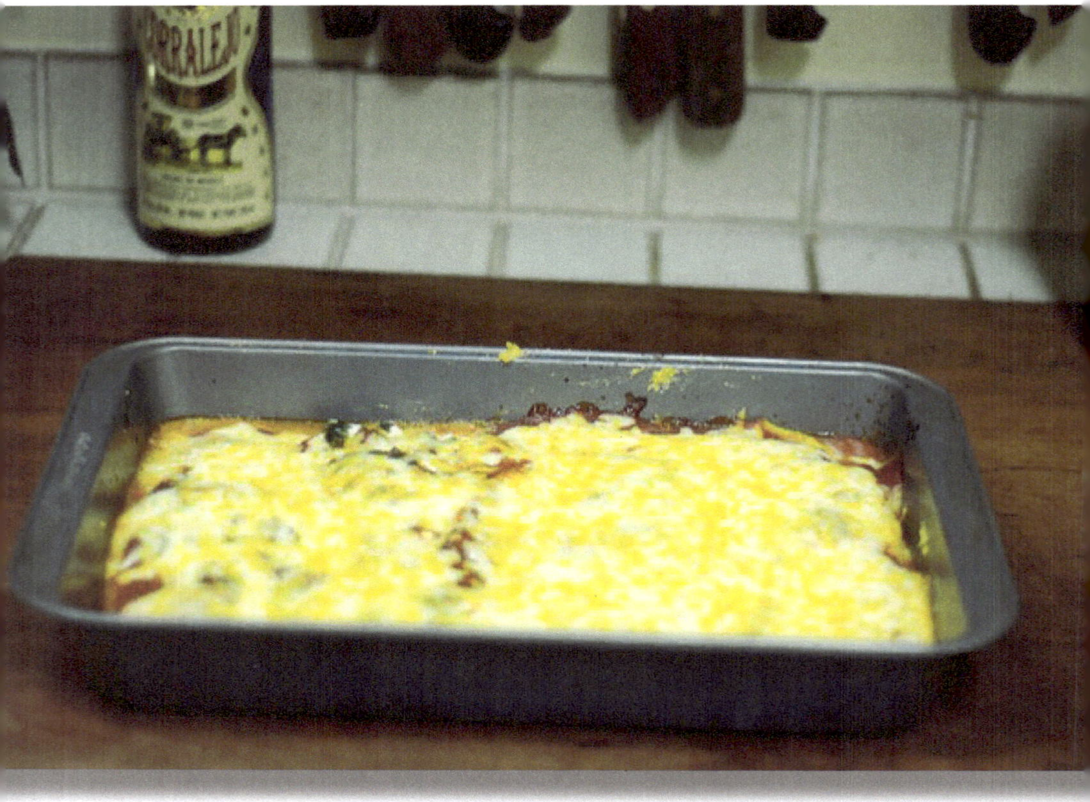

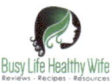

Yummy Polenta Lasagna

Serves: 8   Preparation Time: 10 minutes   Cooking Time: 30 minutes

This flavor-filled, yummy polenta lasagna is a gluten-free, quick, and easy meal for your dinner or lunch.

Ingredients:

- Polenta 1 package (18 ounces)
- Pesto ¼ cup
- Pine nuts ¼ cup
- Marinara sauce ½ jar bottled (24 ounces)
- Mozzarella cheese 1 cup, shredded

Directions:

1. Preheat your oven to 375-degrees F.
2. Grease an 11 by 7 by 2-inch baking dish with oil.
3. In the bottom of the prepared baking dish, arrange a single layer of polenta.
4. Spread a thin layer of pesto over polenta.
5. Then spoon half of the marinara sauce over polenta.
6. Top with another layer of polenta and marinara sauce.
7. Bake for 25 minutes, uncovered.
8. Remove from oven and top with the cheese and pine nuts.
9. Turn on the broiler of your oven and broil the lasagna until cheese is brown and nuts are toasted.

Nutritional Facts Per Serving:

- Calories: 179
- Carbohydrates: 16.7g
- Fats: 9.1g
- Protein: 7.9g

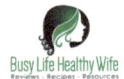

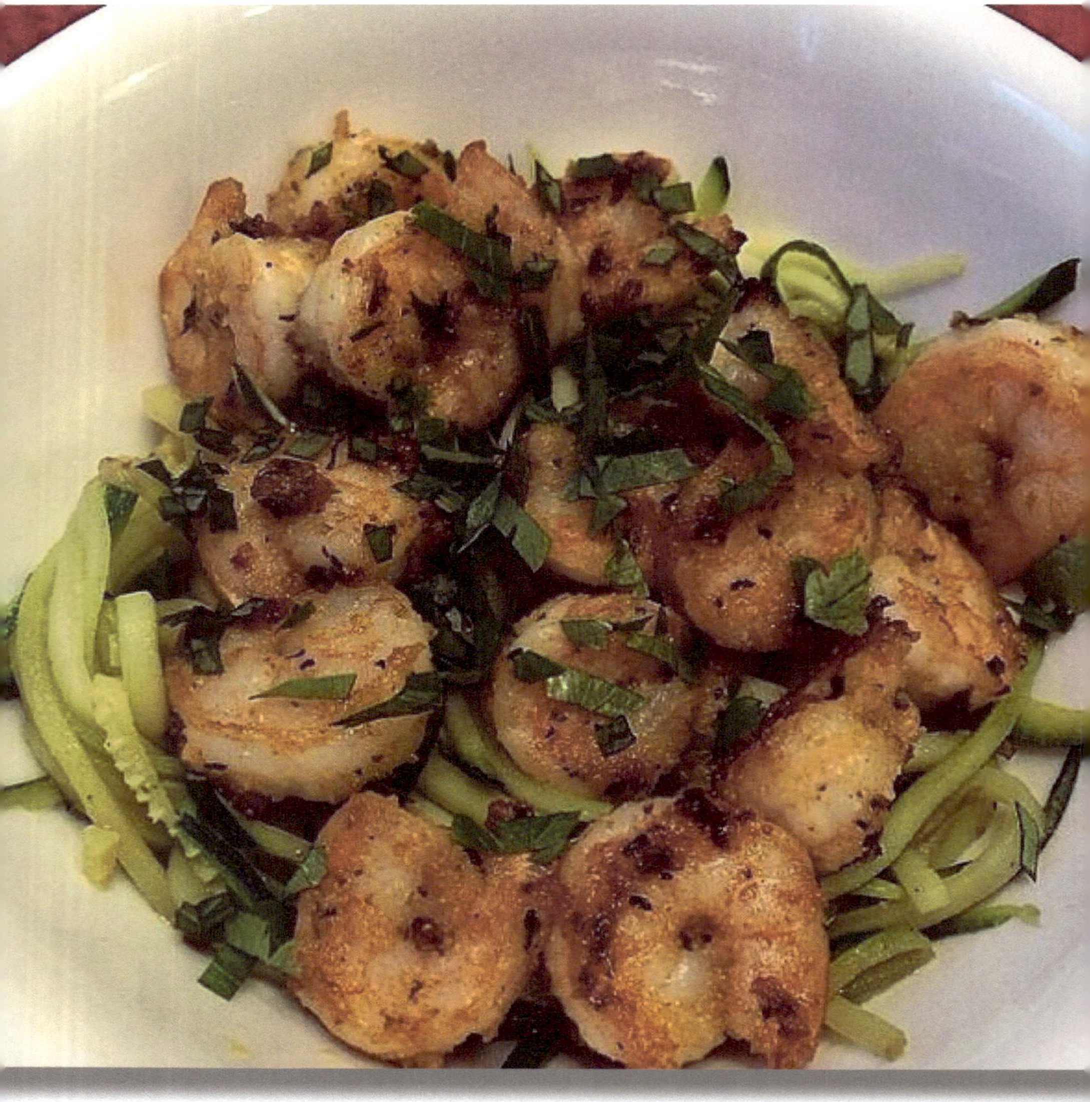

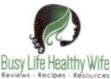

Zoodles with Shrimp

Serves: 4   Preparation Time: 10 minutes   Cooking Time: 15 minutes

To make this dish gluten free, we are using zoodles instead of regular noodles. You can easily make the zucchini noodles with the help of a spiralizer.

Ingredients:

- Large shrimp - 1 pound, peeled and deveined
- Zucchini 2 cut into noodles shape with a spiralizing device
- Baby spinach 1 bag (6 ounces)
- Yellow onion ½ large, minced
- Garlic 1 tablespoon, chopped
- Garlic 1 teaspoon, minced
- Extra virgin olive oil 1 tablespoon
- Butter 3 tablespoons, divided
- Fresh lemon juice 1 tablespoon
- Red pepper flakes 1 teaspoon
- Kosher salt 1 teaspoon, divided
- Freshly ground black pepper ½ teaspoon

Directions:

1. In a large skillet, heat 1 tablespoon butter and olive oil over medium heat.
2. Add zoodles (zucchini noodles), chopped garlic, onion, and ½ teaspoon salt and cook for 5 minutes or until onion is translucent and zoodles are tender.
3. Transfer this zoodles mixture to a bowl.
4. In the same skillet, heat 2 tablespoons butter and add shrimps and minced garlic and cook for 4 minutes or until shrimps are just pink.
5. Stir in lemon juice, spinach, ½ teaspoon salt, red pepper flakes, and black pepper.
6. Cook for 4 minutes more or until spinach begins to wilt.
7. Stir in zoodles mixture and cook for 3 minutes or until heated through.

Nutritional Facts Per Serving:

- Calories: 229
- Carbohydrates: 7.1g
- Fats: 13.4g
- Protein: 21g

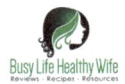

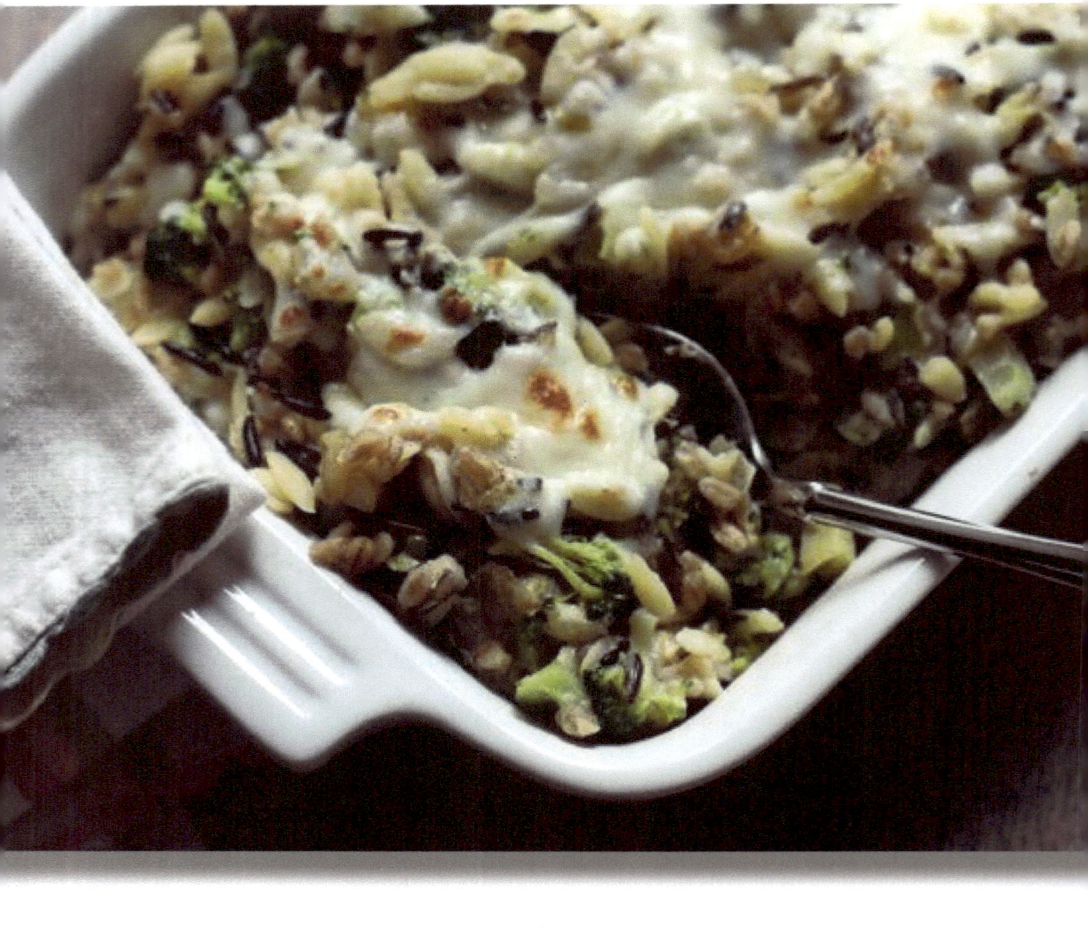

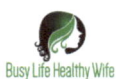

Brown Rice Topped with Broccoli & Oven Toasted Walnuts

Serves: 4   Preparation Time: 15 minutes   Cooking Time: 25 minutes

This tempting dish is surprisingly delicious and flavorful. You can enjoy this gluten-free and healthy meal in your lunch.

Ingredients:

- Uncooked instant brown rice 1 cup
- Fresh broccoli florets 1 pound
- Walnuts ½ cup, chopped
- Homemade vegetable broth 1 cup
- Shredded cheddar cheese 1 cup
- Onion 1 chopped
- Minced garlic ½ teaspoon
- Butter 1 tablespoon
- Salt ½ teaspoon
- Ground black pepper 1/8 teaspoon

Directions:

1. Preheat your oven to 350 degrees F.
2. On a small baking pan, place walnuts and bake for 8 minutes or until toasted.
3. In a medium saucepan, melt butter over medium heat.
4. Add onion and garlic in melted butter and cook for 3 minutes, stirring frequently.
5. Add in the broth and rice, bring it to a boil.
6. Reduce heat to low, cover and simmer for 8 minutes or until liquid is absorbed.
7. Meanwhile, in a microwave safe bowl place broccoli and sprinkle with salt and pepper, cover and microwave until tender.
8. Take a serving platter and spoon rice in it, top rice with broccoli, sprinkle walnuts and cheese on top.
9. Serve immediately.

Nutritional Facts Per Serving:

- Calories: 368
- Carbohydrates: 30.4g
- Fats: 22.9g
- Protein: 15.1g

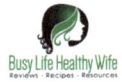

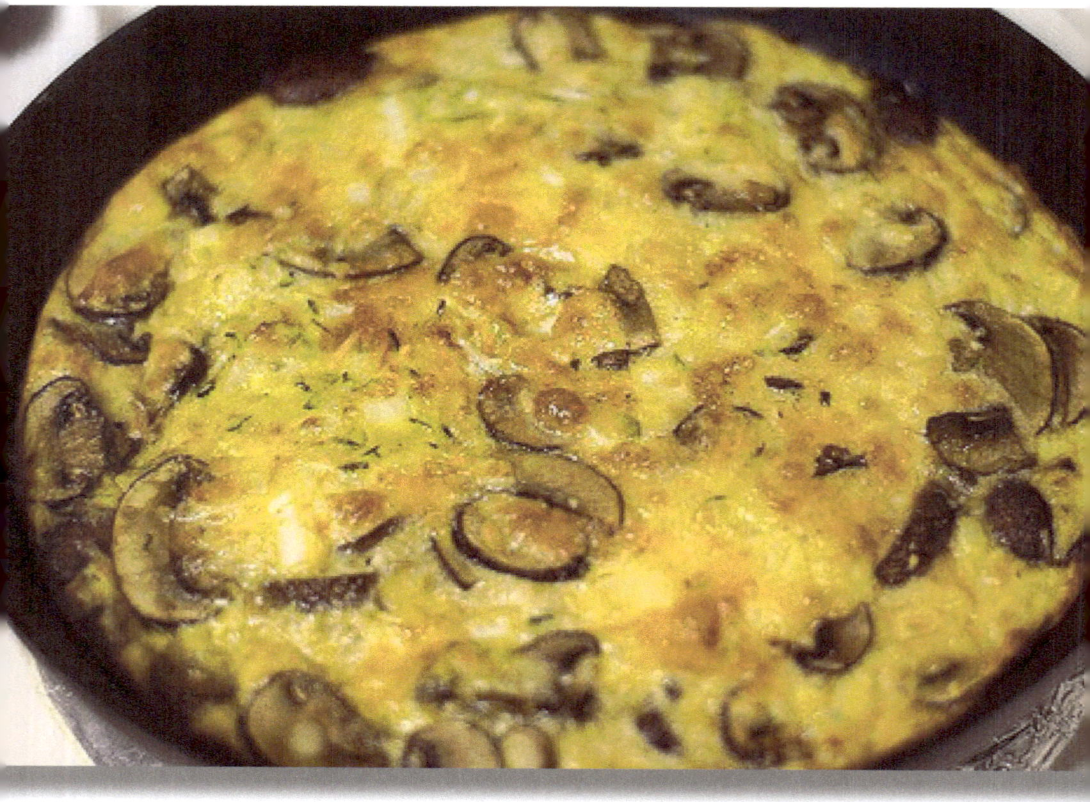

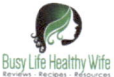

Mushroom Frittata

Serves: 4   Preparation Time: 5 minutes   Cooking Time: 15 minutes

Mushrooms are cooked with scallions and thyme alongside eggs, topped with cheese and baked in a preheated oven.

Ingredients:

- Cremini mushrooms 10 oz, quartered
- Eggs 8 large
- Goat cheese 3 oz
- Extra virgin olive oil 2 tablespoons
- Scallions 2 thinly sliced
- Fresh thyme leaves 2 teaspoons
- Salt and pepper to taste
- Mixed green salad, for serving

Directions:

1. Preheat your oven to 425 degrees F.
2. In a 9-inch cast iron skillet, heat oil over medium-high heat.
3. Add mushrooms to hot oil and cook for 5 minutes or until golden brown.
4. Add in scallions and thyme and cook for 1 minute, stirring continuously.
5. Meanwhile, lightly whisk the eggs in a large bowl, season with salt and pepper.
6. Pour the eggs into the skillet and gently stir, pulling a spatula through the eggs, for 1 minute.
7. Allow it to cook for 1 more minute without stirring.
8. Dollop the goat cheese on top and transfer the skillet to the preheated oven and bake for 8 minutes or until eggs are set.
9. Serve with green salad.

Nutritional Facts Per Serving:

- Calories: 278
- Carbohydrates: 5g
- Fats: 21g
- Protein: 18g

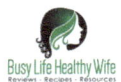

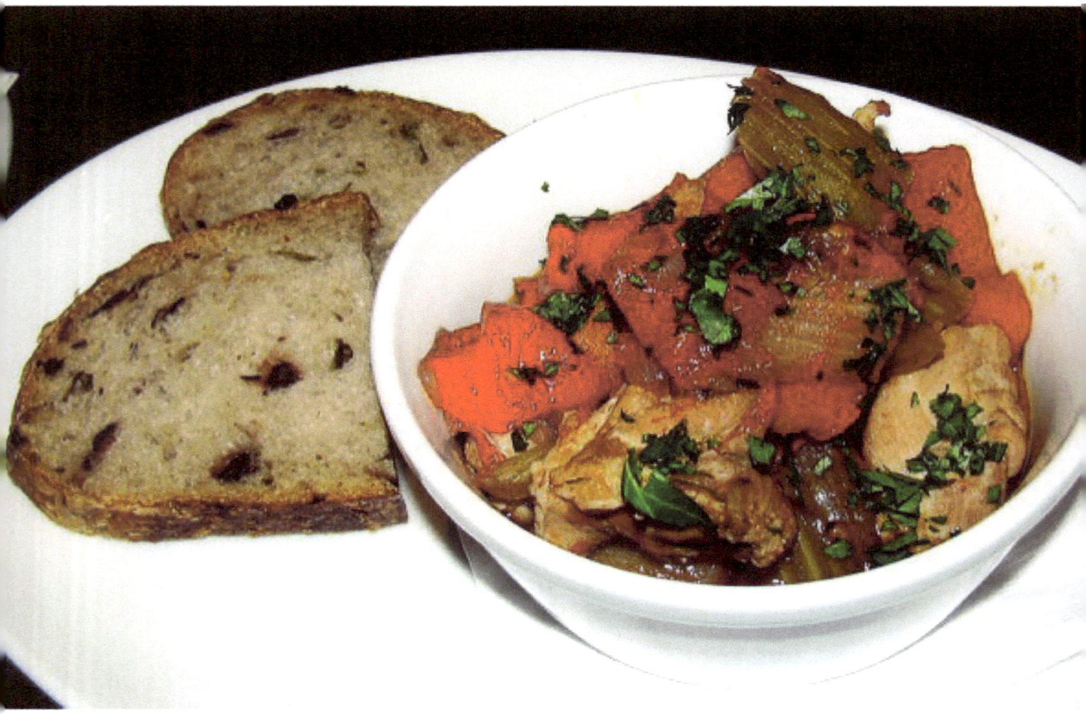

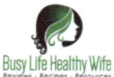

Chicken Cacciatore

Serves: 2   Preparation Time: 5 minutes   Cooking Time: 15 minutes

This is the most simple and classic version of cacciatore. Serve this delicious chicken cacciatore over cooked noodles or rice.

Ingredients:

- Cooked chicken ¾ pound, cubed
- Onion 1/3 cup, chopped
- Green bell pepper 1/3 cup, chopped
- Green beans ½ cup
- Whole peeled tomatoes ½ cup
- Garlic 1 clove, chopped
- Dried oregano ¼ teaspoon

Directions:

1. Sauté onion, garlic, and bell pepper in a large skillet over medium-high heat until soft.
2. Add chicken, then stir in beans, tomatoes, and oregano.
3. Reduce heat low and simmer for 10 minutes, stirring frequently.
4. Remove from heat and serve hot.

Nutritional Facts Per Serving:

- Calories: 240
- Carbohydrates: 8.6g
- Fats: 5.5g
- Protein: 38g

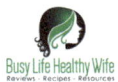

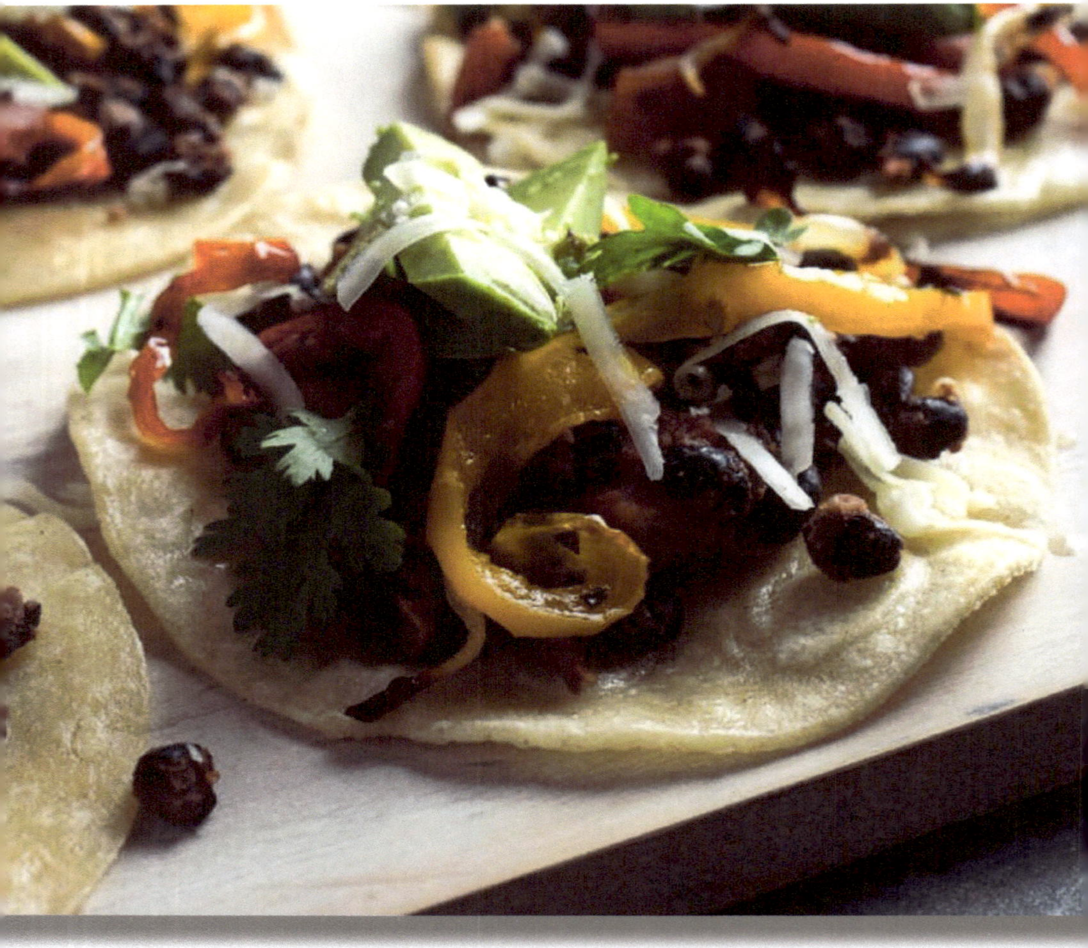

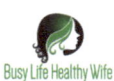

Vegan Fajitas

Serves: 4   Preparation Time: 10 minutes   Cooking Time: 15 minutes

Enjoy your lunch or dinner with these meatless, sweet, and smoky vegan fajitas. Served with corn tortillas to make them gluten free.

Ingredients:

- Corn tortillas 8 small, warmed
- Black bean 1 can (15 oz), rinsed
- Red peppers 2 small, sliced
- Red onion 1 small, thinly sliced
- Pineapple ¼ small, cored and cut into thin pieces
- Chipotles in adobe 1 tablespoon, finely chopped
- Fresh cilantro, for serving
- Sour cream, for serving

Directions:

1. Heat your oven to 425 degrees F.
2. Tear off four 12 inch squares of aluminum foil and arrange on 2 baking sheets.
3. Combine beans and chipotles in a bowl and divide among the 4 pieces of foil.
4. Top with the peppers, pineapple, and onion.
5. Cover with another piece of aluminum foil and fold each edge up and over three times.
6. Roast in preheated oven for 15 minutes.
7. Transfer each packet to a platter.
8. Cut each packet with the knife or scissors and spoon the mixture into tortillas.
9. Top with cilantro and sour cream and serve immediately.

Nutritional Facts Per Serving (1 Fajita):

- Calories: 229
- Carbohydrates: 48g
- Fats: 2g
- Protein: 9g

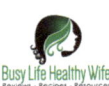

DESSERTS

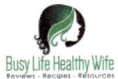

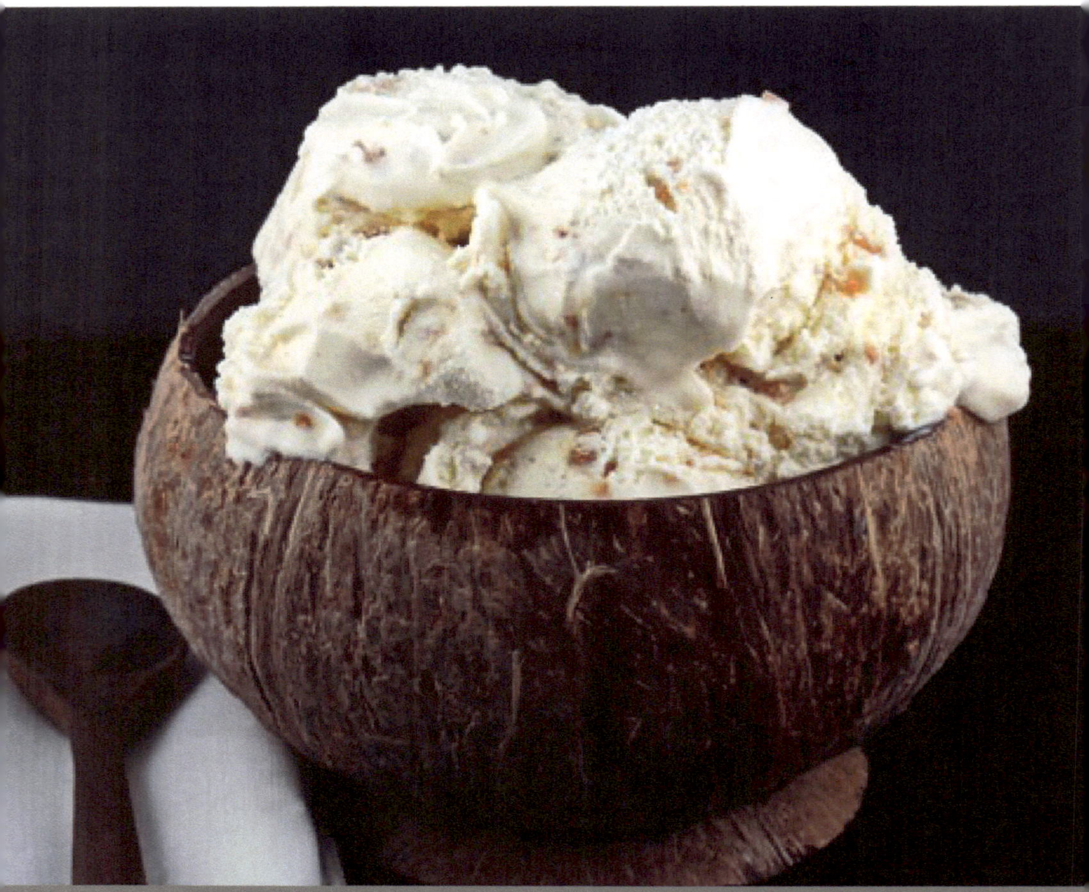

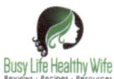

Dairy-Free Coconut Ice

Serves: 12   Preparation Time: 15 minutes

In this dairy free and gluten free coconut ice cream, we have used coconut meat, coconut milk, and bananas.

Ingredients:

- Coconut meat melted ½ cup, such as coconut butter or coconut manna
- "Lite" coconut milk ½ cup
- Very ripe bananas 8
- Unsweetened shredded coconut ¼ cup, toasted, plus more for garnish
- Salt 1 pinch
- Agave syrup ¼ cup

Directions:

1. Peel and slice banana and freeze in an airtight jar for 8 hours or overnight.
2. Combine frozen banana slices, coconut milk, coconut meat, agave, and salt in a food processor and process until smooth.
3. Add in shredded coconut and pulse once or twice just to combine.
4. Immediately serve as soft ice cream or transfer to an airtight container and freeze until firm.
5. To serve scoop into the bowls and garnish with toasted coconut.

Nutritional Facts Per Serving (½ Cup):

- Calories: 171
- Carbohydrates: 26g
- Fats: 8g
- Protein: 2g

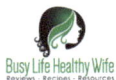

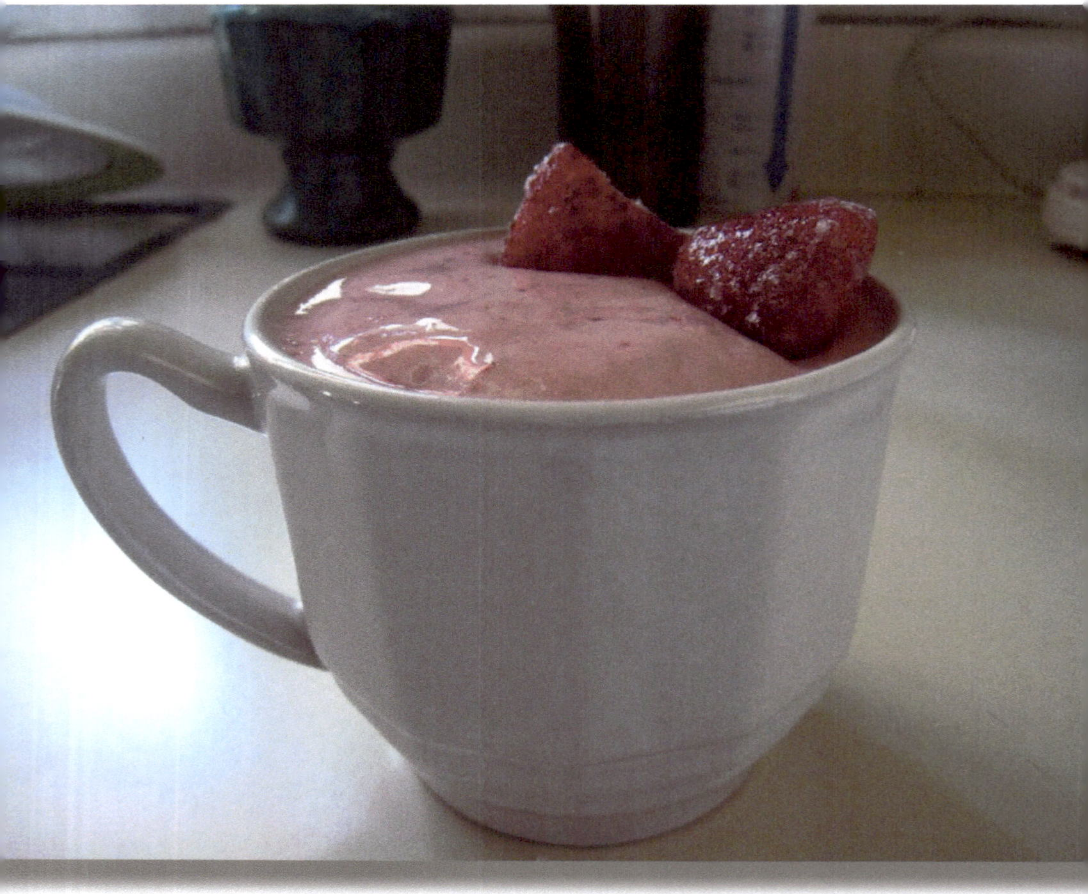

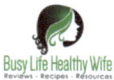

Strawberry Frozen Yogurt

Serves: 4   Preparation Time: 10 minutes

This strawberry frozen yogurt is a great dessert for diabetics and for those on a strict low carb, low calorie, and low-fat diet when made with Greek yogurt as the protein and fiber are generally higher. Additionally, as fruit goes, strawberries have lower carbs.

Ingredients:
- Frozen unsweetened strawberries 1 package (16 ounces)
- Nonfat plain yogurt ½ cup
- Stevia granulated ½ cup
- Lemon juice 1 tablespoon

Directions:
1. Combine strawberries and Stevia in a food processor and process until coarsely chopped.
2. Add lemon juice and yogurt to the food processor and process until smooth and creamy.
3. Serve immediately.

Nutritional Facts Per Serving (3/4 Cup):
- Calories: 58
- Carbohydrates: 13g
- Fats: 0g
- Protein: 2g

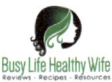

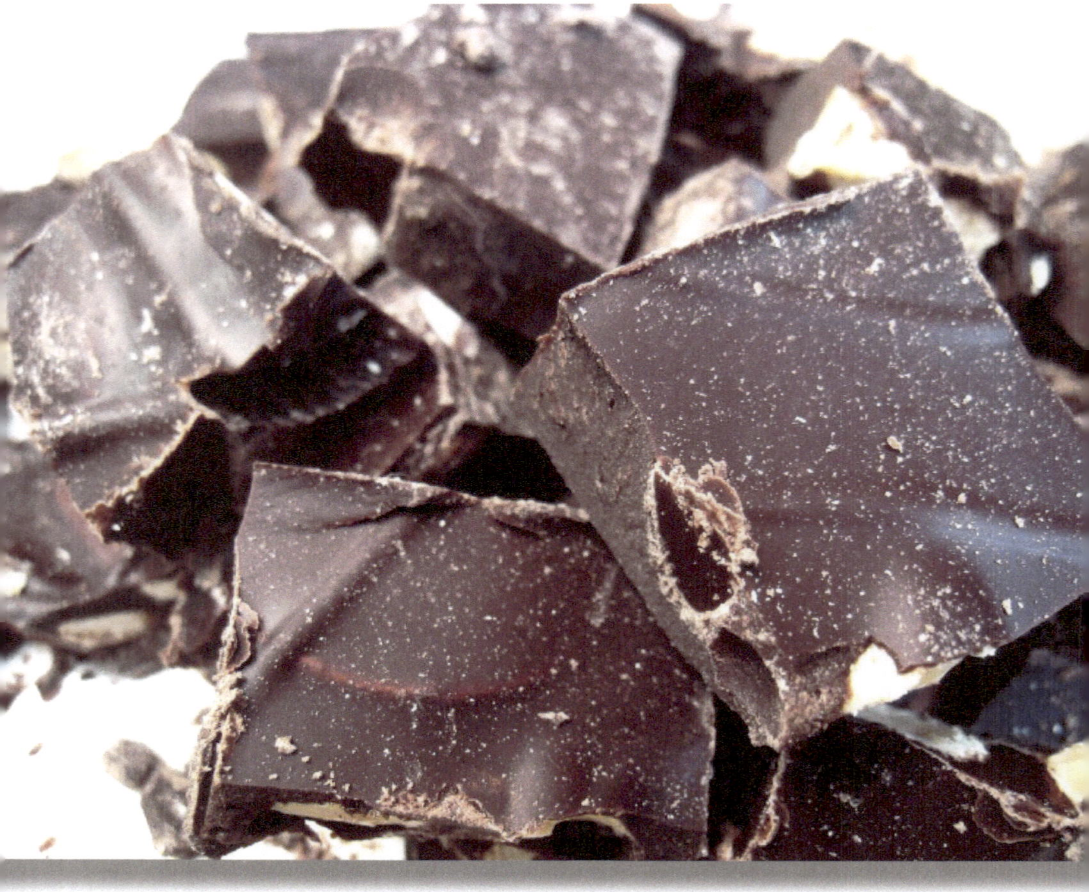

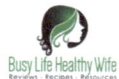

Nutty Chocolate Bar

Serves: 36   Preparation Time: 10 minutes

To make these nutty chocolate bars that are both gluten free and vegan, use your favorite combination of nuts and vegan chocolate.

Ingredients:

- Semi-sweet chocolate 2 cups, melted (or bittersweet or milk chocolate)
- Hazelnut ½ cup
- Almonds ½ cup
- Cashew ½ cup

Directions:

1. Line a rimmed baking sheet with aluminum foil, (take care to avoid wrinkles).
2. Combine hazelnut, almonds, cashews, and melted chocolate in a bowl.
3. Scrape the mixture onto the prepared baking sheet and spread it into an approximate 12 by 9-inch rectangle.
4. Refrigerate for 20 minutes or until set.
5. Transfer the bark with aluminum foil on a clean cutting board.
6. Cut the bark in 1 ½ inch pieces with a sharp knife.
7. Store in an airtight container for up to 2 weeks.

Nutritional Facts Per Serving (1 Piece or 1 ½ Inch):

- Calories: 74
- Carbohydrates: 7g
- Fats: 5g
- Protein: 1g

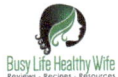

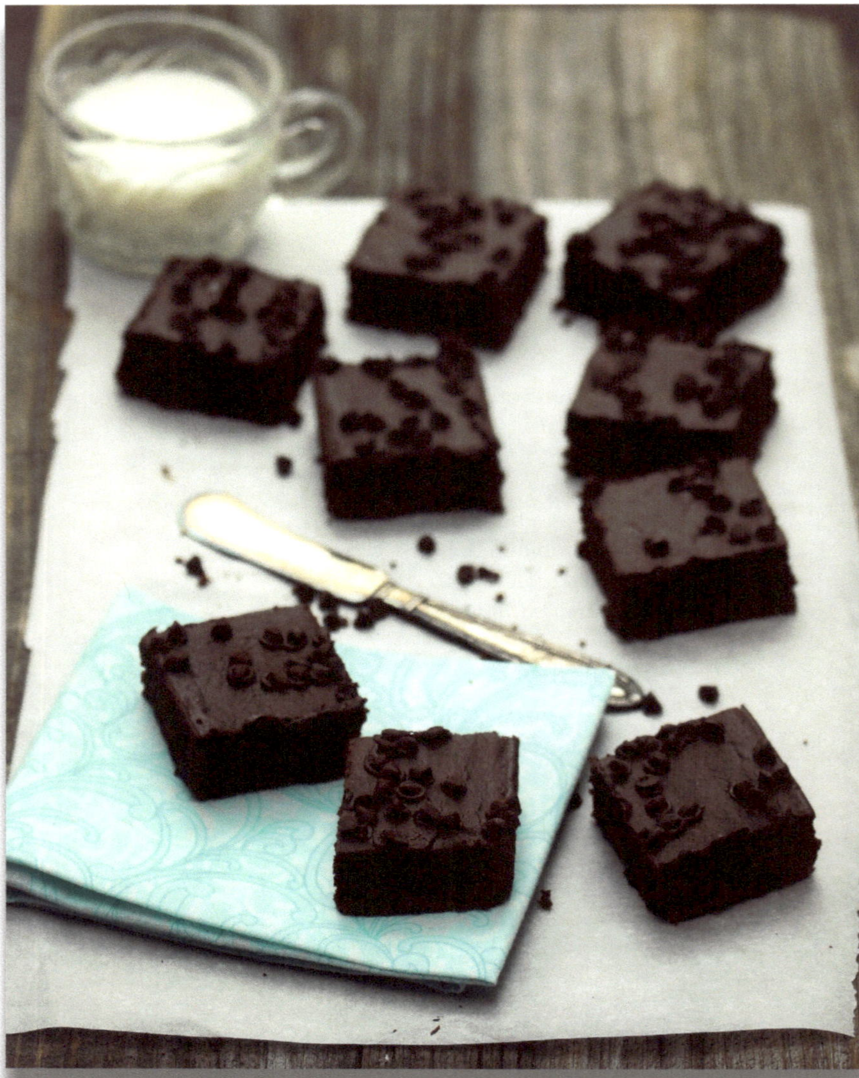

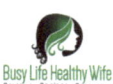

Black Bean Brownie

Serves: 40   Preparation Time: 10 minutes   Cooking Time: 30 minutes

Black beans replace the flour to make this brownie recipe gluten-free, low calorie, healthy, and delicious.

Ingredients:

- Black beans 1 can (15.5 ounces), rinsed and drained
- White sugar ¾ cup
- Cocoa powder ¼ cup
- Milk chocolate chips ½ cup
- Eggs 3
- Vegetable oil 3 tablespoons
- Instant coffee 1 teaspoon
- Vanilla essence 1 teaspoon
- Salt 1 pinch

Directions:

1. Preheat your oven to 350 degrees F.
2. Lightly grease an 8 by 8 square baking dish.
3. Combine all the ingredients except chocolate chips into the blender and blend until smooth.
4. Pour into the prepared baking dish and sprinkle the chocolate chip over the top of the mixture.
5. Bake for 30 minutes or until the top is dry and the edges start to pull away from the sides of the baking pan.

Nutritional Facts Per Serving:

- Calories: 126
- Carbohydrates: 18.1g
- Fats: 5.3g
- Protein: 3.3g

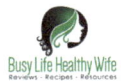

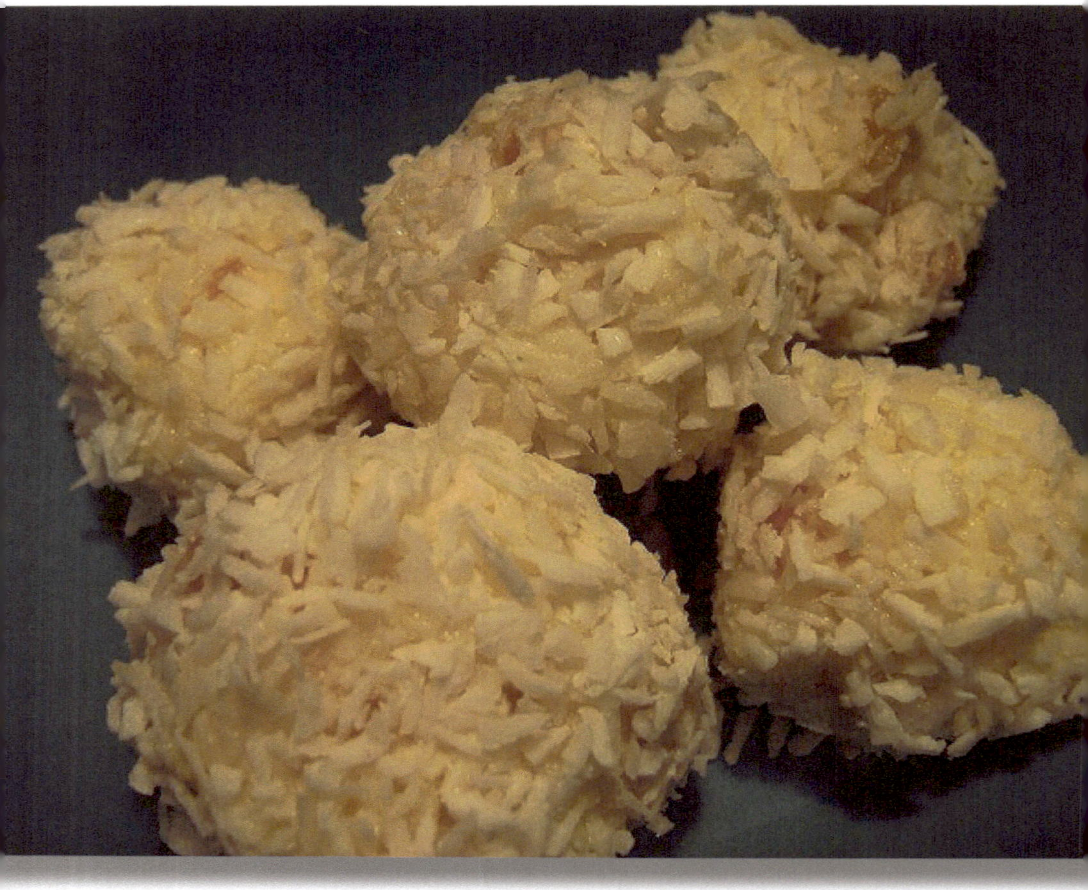

Apricot and Coconut Balls

Serves: 15   Preparation Time: 15 minutes

Dried apricots are minced in a food processor and mixed with flaked coconut, condensed milk, and brown sugar.

Ingredients:
- Dried apricots ½ pound
- Flaked coconut ½ cup
- Brown sugar ½ cup
- Sweetened condensed milk ½ cup (14 ounces)
- Shredded coconut 1 cup, for rolling

Directions:
1. Place dried apricots in a food processor and process until minced.
2. Combine minced apricots, flaked coconut, brown sugar, and condensed milk and mix well.
3. Shape into 1-inch balls and roll in shredded coconut.
4. Refrigerate for at least 40 to 50 minutes and enjoy.

Nutritional Facts Per Serving:
- Calories: 210
- Carbohydrates: 32.5g
- Fats: 9g
- Protein: 2.7g

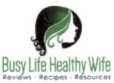

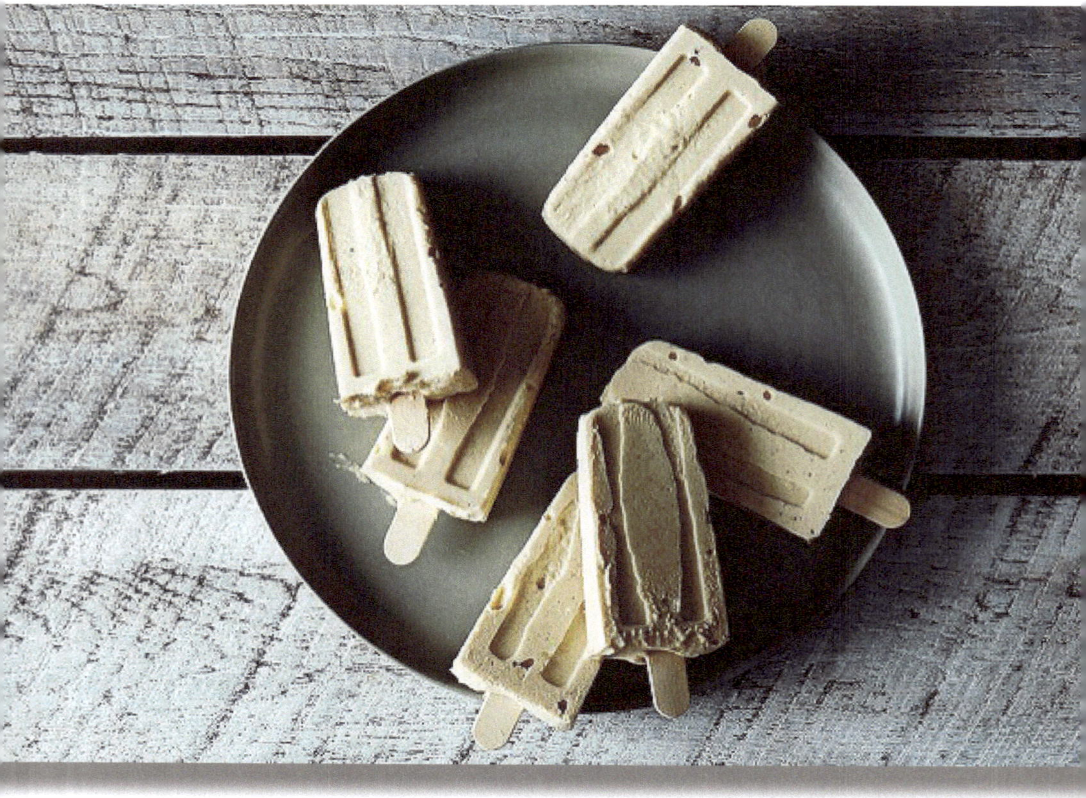

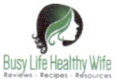

Banana Pudding Pops

Serves: 10   *Preparation Time: 15 minutes*   *Cooking Time: 2 minutes*

These banana pudding pops are really easy to make, gluten free, low fat, and delicious.

Ingredients:

- Bananas 2 large, diced (2 cups)
- Low-fat milk 2 cups
- Light brown sugar ½ cup
- Cornstarch 2 tablespoons
- Vanilla essence 2 teaspoons
- Salt 1 pinch
- Popsicle molds 1 set

Directions:

1. To make pudding, in a large saucepan whisk together milk, cornstarch, brown sugar, and salt until combined.
2. Heat over medium-high heat and bring it to a boil, whisking continuously.
3. Boil for 1 minute and remove from heat and stir in vanilla essence.
4. Transfer half of the pudding in a food processor and add bananas, process until smooth.
5. Stir this blended mixture into the remaining ½ of the pudding.
6. Evenly divide the mixture among freezer pop molds.
7. Freeze for 1 hour remove from freezer insert sticks and put it back in the freezer for at least 6 hours or overnight.

Nutritional Facts Per Serving (1 Pop):

- Calories: 80
- Carbohydrates: 17g
- Fats: 1g
- Protein: 2g

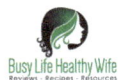

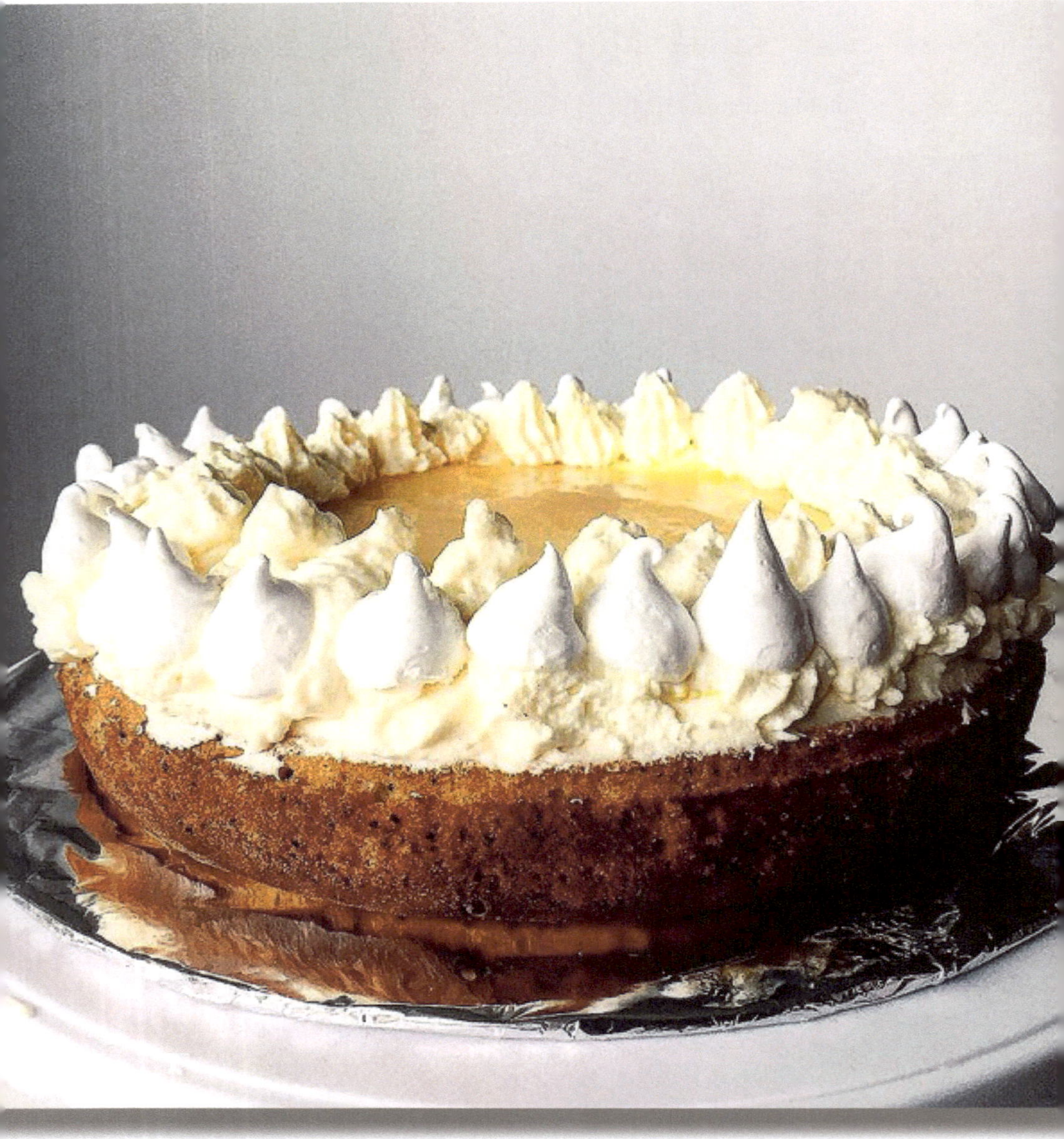

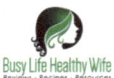

Gluten-Free Cake

Serves: 24   Preparation Time: 10 minutes   Cooking Time: 25 minutes

This is the basic recipe of a gluten-free cake; you can frost it with any of your favorite gluten-free frostings, top it with fruit, or add powdered sugar to it. To make the cake extra moist and delicious, replace one egg with one heaping tablespoons of plain or vanilla regular or Greek yogurt.

Ingredients

- White rice flour 1 ½ cups
- White sugar 1 ¼ cups
- Tapioca flour ¾ cup
- Baking powder 3 teaspoons
- Baking soda 1 teaspoon
- Xanthan gum 1 teaspoon
- Salt 1 teaspoon
- Eggs 4
- Milk 1 cup
- Mayonnaise 2/3 cup
- Gluten-free vanilla essence 2 teaspoons
- 8-inch round cake pans 2

Directions:

1. Preheat your oven to 350 degrees F.
2. Grease and rice flour 2 eight-inch round cake pans.
3. Combine rice flour, tapioca flour, baking powder, baking soda, xanthan gum, and salt in a bowl and mix well.
4. In a large mixing bowl, whisk the eggs, mayonnaise, and sugar until fluffy.
5. Add the flour mixture, vanilla essence, and milk in the egg mixture and mix well.
6. Divide the batter in both prepared cake pans.
7. Bake for 25 minutes or until a toothpick inserted in the center of the cake comes out clean.
8. Let it cool for 10 minutes in the pan then remove from the pan.

Nutritional Facts Per Serving:

- Calories: 154
- Carbohydrates: 23.1g
- Fats: 6g
- Protein: 2.1g

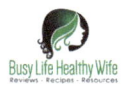

Thank You

Thank you again for purchasing **A Cookbook for Busy Lives: 30 Healthy, Gluten Free Recipes.**

Did you make one of these recipes or a different gluten free recipe for your friends, yourself, or your family? I'd love to see your photos and videos of you creating the dish, finalizing it, or sharing it with others. With your permission, I may even feature your content on one of my social media channels or ***www.busylifehealthywife.com.***

If you would like to be updated on upcoming cookbooks and other health, productivity, and life hacks, sign up for the "Healthy Habit Herald Newsletter" on ***busylifehealthywife.com.***

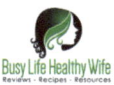

www.ingramcontent.com/pod-product-compliance
Lightning Source LLC
Chambersburg PA
CBHW041220070526
44584CB00001B/22